PSYCHIATRY - THEORY, APPLICATIONS AND TREATMENTS

ADHD

VARIABILITY BETWEEN MIND AND BODY

PSYCHIATRY - THEORY, APPLICATIONS AND TREATMENTS

Additional books in this series can be found on Nova's website under the Series tab.

Additional e-books in this series can be found on Nova's website under the e-book tab.

PSYCHIATRY - THEORY, APPLICATIONS AND TREATMENTS

ADHD

VARIABILITY BETWEEN MIND AND BODY

RADEK PTACEK, PHD
AND
HANA KUZELOVA, PHD

New York

Library of Congress Cataloging-in-Publication Data

ISBN: 978-1-63321-449-1

Library of Congress Control Number: 2014959222

Published by Nova Science Publishers, Inc. † New York

Contents

Introduction

The diagnostic category of Attention-Deficit/Hyperactivity Disorder (ADHD) became a distinct phenomenon in research and clinical practice in the last decades. Additionally, the disorder is no longer solely isolated within the field of psychiatry. Implementing the category intended to provide a greater definition as well as overarching clarity about minimal brain dysfunctions and related concepts that were rather vague. It is apparent that our current clinical practice and research involving this new concept brings about more questions than answers. However, despite fevered discussions regarding the diagnosis of ADHD, it is more apparent that the problems associated with it are not limited to psychiatry but also cover psychological, social and possibly psychosomatic developments.

ADHD is one of the most commonly diagnosed disorders in childhood today. ADHD is characterized as a group of developmental disorders that includes a combination of hyperactivity, impulsivity, and inattention. The disorder manifests itself during the child's development by debilitating cognitive, executive, and perceptual-motoric functions. Additional affected areas are indicated through decreased ability to regulate affection, emotivism, and social adaptability.

In a sense, ADHD clearly illustrates interaction among genetic, neurobiological, and epigenetic factors. The causes of ADHD are not yet fully understood but the greatest indicators are attributed to heredity and biological factors (i.e. abnormal fetal development, developmental impairments, etc.). Existing studies show that especially dysfunctional genes in dopamine receptors, dopamine, and serotonin transporters contribute towards the development of ADHD. However, others genes are believed to be involved as well as the contribution of environmental factors that play an important role in the evolution of ADHD.

ADHD is also accompanied by neuroendocrinological changes that when combined with other changes foster discussions about possible discrepancies in growth and physical development of the individual inflicted with ADHD. Based on available study results, children with ADHD have decreased body growth, but tend to have a higher Body Mass Index (BMI) and proportion of fat deposits in the body tissue. [213, 211, 214] These changes can also result from specific differences in eating habits – e.g. impulsivity when consuming food and preference for fast food. [66] Higher incidence of obesity in patients with ADHD can also result from greater difficulties they experience with weight reduction that is caused by lowered self-control. [2, 71]

Diagnosing adults with ADHD did not appear until the Diagnostic and Statistical Manual of Mental Disorders 5th revision (DSM-5) was published in May 2013. In previous versions, ADHD was primarily diagnosed in children and in lesser cases adolescents. All previous medical recommendations and diagnostic procedures were primarily related to the fields of child psychiatry and psychology. From this point on the view on ADHD changed and today the defining characteristics of ADHD have expanded beyond traditional bounds into adults. Additionally, based on a number of empirical and clinical research findings, ADHD is viewed as a disorder that pervades throughout the entire life of an individual, which allows for its diagnosis and treatment at all stages of human life.

ADHD is a disorder with exceptional variability in many respects, such as causes, manifestations, development, and response to treatment. Some individuals are genetically predisposed but do not exhibit symptoms of ADHD, while others do. ADHD may have quite a negative impact on the bearer's ability to adapt to life and their overall quality of life is likely to be diminished. Other individuals will have no life hindering effects associated with the diagnosis. Thus, ADHD poses many exceptions and is by no means a simple diagnosis. Any diagnosis is only an effort to categorize variable groups of causes and manifestations.

The presented book is based on previous research and review work of authors and is the English version of the book published in the Czech language [210]. It provides a complex and comprehensive insight into problems with variability of ADHD – from etiology to neurobiology and somatic causes through psychological and social contexts. The aim of this publication is not to present an elaborate and detailed analysis of the particular circumstances but to provide more general overview of the attributes associated with ADHD. The basic feature of ADHD is its variability, which is characteristic for all symptoms related with this disorder. Variability is also the central concept and basis of this publication. It is our hope that we do not just offer new information, but an alternate view on the phenomenon that is often considered one of the primary themes in psychiatry and psychology in the 21st century.

The book is supported by the project "PRVOUK PSYCHOLOGIE - P03/LF1/9"

Radek Ptacek
Hana Kuzelova
Department of Psychiatry First Faculty of Medicine Charles University in Prague and General University Hospital in Prague

List of Acronyms

AAP	American Academy of Pediatrics
ACTH	Adrenocorticotropic hormone
ADD	Attention Deficit Disorder
ADHD	Attention-Deficit/Hyperactivity Disorder
ADHD-C	Attention-Deficit/Hyperactivity Disorder Combined Type – Combined type
ADHD-I	Attention-Deficit/Hyperactivity Disorder Inattentive Type – Inattentive type
ADHD-HI	Attention-Deficit/Hyperactivity Disorder Hyperactive/ Impulsive Type – Hyperactive/Impulsivetype
ADRA2A	Alpha-2-adrenergic receptor
Amx	Atomoxetine
BMI	Body Mass Index
BMR	Basal metabolism
NAR	National anthropological research
CBCL	Child Behavior Checklist
CPQ	Conners Parents Questionnaire
CD	Conduct disorders
CT	Computed tomography
COMT	Catechol-O-methyl transferase
DAT	Dopamine transporter
DAT1	Gene for dopamine transporter
Dex	Dextroamfetamine
DBH	Dopamine beta-hydroxylase
DNA	Deoxyribonucleicacid
DRD	Genefor dopamine receptor

DSM-IV	Diagnostic and Statistical Manual of Mental Disorders 4th revision
EEG	Electroencephalography
fMRI	Functional Magnetic Resonance Imaging
GABA	Gama-Aminobutyric acid
GH	Growth hormone
GIT	Gastrointestinal tract
HPA axis	Hypothalamic-pituitary-adrenal axis
HTR1B	5-hydroxytryptamine receptor 1B
HT	Hydroxytryptamine
ICD-10	International Classification of Diseases
IQ	Intelligencequotient
CBT	Cognitive-behavioral therapy
LBD	Light brain dysfunction
MAO	Monoamine oxidases
MAO-A	Monoamine oxidases A
MKN-10	International Classification of Diseases, 10th revision
Mph	Methylphenidate
MRI	Magnetic Resonance Imaging
ODD	Oppositional defiant disorder
PDD	Pervasive developmental disorder
SDS	SD score
SNAP25	Synaptosomal-associated protein 25
SNP	Single Nucleotide Polymorphism
T3	Triiodothyronine
T4	Thyroxine
TACR1	Tachykinin receptor 1
TRH	Thyrotropin-releasing hormone
VNTR	Variable number of tandem repeat
WHO	World Health Organization
5-HT	5-hydroxytryptamine receptor, Serotonin
5-HTT	Serotonin transporter

Chapter 1

Concept Evolution, Diagnosis and Etiology of ADHD

Abstract

The chapter provides basic information about the evolution of therminology of diagnosis of ADHD. The diagnostic criteria according to DSM-IV, DSM-5 are presented here and compared with ICD-10. The chapter provides also information about differential diagnostics, because many symptoms of ADHD can be also observed in other diagnoses, therefore ADHD is comorbid with other psychiatric disorders. The most common comorbid diagnoses are discussed here. Then etiology of ADHD is briefly metioned in this chapter, however e.g. biological (mainly genetical) connections are subject of following chapters. This chapter also provides information about the prevalence of ADHD and its manifestation across the lifespan.

1.1. Concept Evolution and Criteria of ADHD

Professional terminology in the field of hyperactivity and attention disorders has undergone a number of changes throughout its history. The developmental timeline of ADHD shows us different concepts that reflect the perceived etiology of the disease. Early beliefs relied upon organic causes, such as *minimal brain damage*. Later studies are tending to focus on dominant behavioral manifestations, such as *hyperkinetic syndrome, hyperexcitable syndrome*, etc. Conceptual understanding of problems with minimal developmental disorders, have evolved, illustrating the shift from highlighting the cause of a diagnosis (*minimal brain damage)* towards evaluating individual characteristics (*Attention Deficit Disorder*).

The first known documented description of today's ADHD behavioral characteristics was recorded in 1902 when George Still, a British physician gave a lecture about *abnormal defects of moral control* in a group of children. [257] These children supposedly showed weak self-control, excessive motor activity and impatience. He described his findings as an abnormal defect of moral control with want on mischievousness and destructiveness. [257] In the following years numerous diagnostic and descriptive terms appeared in records describing the disorder presently known as ADHD:

- The first systematic description available under the name *brain disorders* originated in the 1940's. During this time the main focus was on the organic cause of the brain disorder. The main organic causes that were identified were structural brain abnormalities, current impairments of the central nervous system, and excessive or insufficient stimulation. [122]
- 1937: Dr. Charles Bradley published results of his study about children with *organic brain syndrome*. The use of Benzedrine to treat these children improved their behavior and school performance (dextroamphetamine sulfate). [41]
- 1947: the disorder is recognized as a result of *brain damage* (Strauss and Lehtinen) or *Minimal Brain Damage*. (Gessel and Amatruda). [258, 105]
- 1952: First publication of the Diagnostic and statistical manual used terminology of *Minimal Brain Dysfunction* (MBD) and *Hyperkinetic syndrom*e. [6]
- 1957: *"Hyperkinetic impulse disorder*" attributed symptoms to excessive cortisol stimulation. [155] The field begins to reference *"Cerebral Dysfunctions*" with the focus shifting towards specific developmental impairments in academic skills.
- 1960: *"Hyperactive Child Syndrome" focused* on excessive motor activity. [58]
- 1968: DSM-II used the concept "*Hyperkinetic Reaction of Childhood*" (or adolescence) and made it very that if existing symptoms are

secondary to the organic brain damage, it should not be used in a diagnosis (APA). [7] This DSM version also included symptoms of inattention, short attention span, over activity and restlessness.

- In the 1970's and 1980's the emphasis aimed toward the identification of the most prominent manifestations of the disorder, such as restlessness and elevated activity levels. [21]
- 1980: DSM-III used the concepts "*Attention Deficit Disorder with Hyperactivity*" (ADDH), *"Attention Deficit Disorder"* (ADD), and "*Attention Deficit Disorder - Residual Type*" (ADD-RT) (APA). [8] ADDH gives equal weight to three areas of the disorder: inattention, impulsivity, and hyperactivity. ADD combines inattention and impulsivity with a possible absence of hyperactivity. ADD-RT takes into account residual symptoms that persist after hyperactivity subsided.
- 1987: DSM-III-R combines the symptoms into a single list under one diagnostic category ***"Attention-Deficit/Hyperactive Disorder" (ADHD)***. [9] Additionally, other symptoms of hyperactivity were added within this category. A new concept was introduced indicating that existing symptoms exhibited by a patient must be more prominent than the symptoms exhibited by the "*majority of population of the same mental age*". [9, s. 52] "Undifferentiated ADD" was included within a special section of the manual DSM-III-R and contained symptoms of inattention.
- 1994: DSM-IV identifies so called subtypes of ADHD – ***"Predominantly Inattentive Type, Predominantly Hyperactive-Impulsive Type, and Combined Type"*** (APA). [10] The diagnostic category ***"Not Otherwise Specified ADHD"*** was also included in the manual.
- 2013: DSM-5 (APA, American Psychiatric Association) follows the basic concept of ADHD according to DSM-IV but ADHD is presented as whole-life diagnosis and the criteria are changed according to this fact. [12]

1.2. Diagnosis of ADHD

1.2.1. Criteria in DSM-IV

In the last decade, the DSM-IV significantly influenced the manner in which a diagnosis of ADHD was derived. The clinical and scientific fields fully accepted the diagnostic criteria of ADHD which considerably influenced the overall approach to diagnostics, treatment, and research of the disorder. The concept of the disorder is understood mostly as a developmental disorder and its criteria are associates only with children. The DSM-5 later changed the application of the criteria to include the diagnosis and treatment of ADHD in adults.

In the revision of the DSM-IV, ADHD is categorized under *"Disorders usually first diagnosed in infancy, childhood, or adolescence"* (DSM-IV-TR; APA). [11] Behavioral criteria are divided into three categories: *Inattention, Hyperactivity, and Impulsivity.* Nine criteria in the diagnostic category "Inattention" include the primary problems with attention (e.g., failure to give close attention to details) and secondary effects of inattention (e.g., losing necessary things). Nine criteria in the diagnostic category "Hyperactivity" and "Impulsivity" contain motoric (e.g., fidgeting with hands or feet) as well as verbal manifestations (e.g., blurt out the answer without thinking). All of these 18 symptoms contain the word "often" which indicates a diagnosis of ADHD is not warranted when the symptoms appear only on an occasional basis.

In order to be diagnosed, children and adolescents must meet the following criteria at specific ages; disorder manifestation, visible maladaptation, and repetitive patterns of behavior. Certain symptoms of ADHD must be observed before 7 years of age, even though the full manifestation of the disorder is not fully apparent. These symptoms must continue to be persistent, i.e. must be present in at least two settings (e.g., at school, at home, and other areas of society) and must be inconsistent with the developmental level (at least 6 months). Furthermore, symptoms must be clinically assessable changes in normal daily functioning in order to fall within the diagnostic parameters of ADHD.

Symptoms must be **maladaptive and inconsistent with the developmental level of a child.** For example, a 13 years old child with an apparent normal developmental level and average intelligence that displays attention deficiencies and impaired behavioral control may be suffering from ADHD. On the other hand, if another 13 years old child displays the same intellectual and cognitive abilities of a 6 year old and is not displaying consistent developmental levels with other normal 13 years olds, a diagnosis of ADHD is not entirely eliminated but is generally not justified.

The DSM-IV-TR indicates other disorders with some of the symptoms similar to ADHD must be considered as well. For example, Pervasive Developmental Disorder (PDD), Schizophrenia, Other Psychotic Disorders, Mood Disorders, Anxiety Disorders, Dissociative Disorder, and Personality Disorder.

The main characteristics of ADHD as described in the DSM-IV-TR are **inattention, hyperactivity,** and/or **impulsivity**. These characteristics must also contain the following criteria:

- Must be present often
- Must be present before age 7
- Must be persistent (consistent)
- Must be pervasive (occur in all settings)
- Must be inconsistent with the development level
- Must cause maladaptation
- Can not meet the criteria of another diagnosis

1.2.2. Criteria in DSM-5

The DSM-5 brings new understanding of ADHD just as the DSM-IV did when first introduced (APA). [12] ADHD is no longer considered a developmental disorder, but is now a disorder that can manifest itself throughout the entire life of an individual. However, the onset of ADHD still remains consistent with the previous manuals assessment that the disorder originates in childhood. The DSM-5 redefined the age parameters for symptoms to be present before the age of 12 rather than the DSM-IV definition of symptoms being present before the age of 7. The primary characteristics of ADHD in DSM-5 are still persistent inattention and/or hyperactivity-impulsivity that affect the normal functioning of an individual and his or her performance in life.

The DSM-5 defines three main types of ADHD as a combined presentation, predominantly inattentive representation and predominantly hyperactive/impulsive presentation. The DSM-5 also defines three levels of severity: mild, moderate, and severe, that are assessed based on impairment in social, academic, and occupational functioning. The category "partial remission" is also defined in the DSM-5 and is being used when the full criteria previously met and when fewer than full criteria are met during the last few months but the symptoms are still causing impairments in social, academic, or occupational functioning.

Diagnostic Criteria

A. Persistent pattern of inattention and/or hyperactivity-impulsivity that interferes with functioning or development, as characterized by (1) or (2):

1. **Inattention:** Six or more of the following symptoms must have persisted for at least 6 months to a degree that is inconsistent with developmental level and that negatively impacts directly on social and academic/occupational activities:

   Note. The symptoms are not solely a manifestation of oppositional behavior, defiance, hostility, or failure to understand tasks or instructions. For older adolescents and adults (age 17 and older), at least five symptoms are required.

   a. Often fails to give close attention to details or makes careless mistakes in schoolwork, at work, or during other activities (e.g., overlooks or misses details, work is inaccurate).
   b. Often has difficulty sustaining attention in tasks or play activities (e.g., has difficulty remaining focused during lectures, conversations, or lengthy reading).
   c. Often does not seem to listen when spoken directly (e.g., mind seems elsewhere, even in the absence of any obvious distraction).
   d. Often does not follow through on instructions a fails to finish schoolwork, chores, or duties in the workplace (e.g., starts tasks quickly but loses focus and is easily sidetracked).
   e. Often has difficulty organizing tasks and activities (e.g., difficulty managing sequential tasks; difficulty keeping materials and belongings in order; messy, disorganized work; poor time management; fails to meet deadlines).
   f. Often avoids or dislikes tasks that require sustained mental effort (e.g., schoolwork or homework; for older adolescents and adults, preparing reports, completing forms, reviewing lengthy papers).
   g. Often loses things necessary for tasks or activities (e.g., school materials, pencils, books, wallets, keys, paperwork, eyeglasses, mobile phones).

h. Is often easily distracted by extraneous stimuli (for older adolescents and adults, may include unrelated thoughts).
i. Is often forgetful in daily activities (e.g., doing chores, running errands; for older adolescents and adults, returning calls, paying bills, keeping appointments).

2. **Hyperactivity and impulsivity:**

Six or more of the following symptoms have persisted for at least 6 months to a degree that is inconsistent with developmental level and that negatively impacts directly on social and academic/occupational activities:

Note. These symptoms are not solely a manifestation of oppositional behavior, defiance, hostility, or a failure to understand tasks or instructions. For older adolescents and adults (age 17 and older), at least five symptoms are required:

a. Often fidgets with or taps hands or feet or squirms in seat.
b. Often leaves seat in situations when remaining seated is expected (e.g., leaves his or her place in the classroom, in the office or the workplace, or in other situations that require remaining in place).
c. Often runs about or climbs in situations where it is inappropriate (Note: In adolescents or adults, may be limited to feeling restless.).
d. Often unable to play or engage in leisure activities quietly.
e. Is often "on the go", acting as if "driven by a motor" (e.g., is unable to be or uncomfortable being still for extended time, as in restaurants, meetings; may be experienced by others as being restless or difficult to keep up with).
f. Often talks excessively.
g. Often blurts out an answer before a question has been completed (e.g., completes people's sentences; can not wait for turn in conversation).
h. Often has difficulty to wait for his or her turn (e.g., while waiting in line).
i. Often interrupts or intrudes on others (e.g., butts into conversations, games, or activities; may start using others people's things without asking or receiving permission; for adolescents and adults, may intrude into or take over what others are doing).

B. Several inattentive or hyperactive-impulsive symptoms were present prior to age 12 years.

C. Several inattentive or hyperactive-impulsive symptoms are present in two or more settings (e.g., at home, school, or work; with friends or relatives; in other activities).

D. There is clear evidence that the symptoms interfere with, or reduce the quality of, social, academic, or occupational functioning.

E. The symptoms do not occur exclusively during the course of schizophrenia or another psychotic disorder and are not better explained by another mental disorder (e.g., affective disorder, anxiety disorder, dissociative disorder, personality disorder, substance intoxication or withdrawal).

Specify whether:

314.01 (F90.2) Combined presentation disorder: If both criteria A1 (inattention) and A2 (hyperactivity-impulsivity) are met for the past 6 moths.

314.00 (F90.0) Predominantly inattentive disorder: If Criterion A1 (inattention) is met but Criterion A2 (hyperactivity-impulsivity) is not met for the past 6 months.

314.01 (F90.1) Predominantly hyperactive/impulsive disorder: If Criterion A2 (hyperactivity-impulsivity) is met but Criterion A1 (inattention) is not met for the past 6 months.

Specify, if:

In partial remission: when full criteria were previously met, fewer than the full criteria have been met for the past 6 months, and the symptoms still result in impairment in social, academic, or occupational functioning.

Specify current severity:

Mild: few, if any, symptoms in excess of those required to make a diagnosis are present, and symptoms result in no more than minor impairments in social or occupational functioning.

Moderate: symptoms or functional impairment between "mild" and "severe" are present.

Severe: many symptoms in excess of those required to make diagnosis, or several symptoms that are particularly severe are present, or the symptoms result in marked impairment in social or occupational functioning.

1.2.3. International Classification of Diseases ICD -10

"International Statistical Classification of Diseases and Health Related Problems“ is an international medical reference used in the field of clinical medicine (ICD-10). The ICD manual originated from a document in the 1900's and is regularly revised at international conferences organized by the World Health Organization (WHO). The ICD is used to monitor mortality rates (e.g., cause of death relative to diagnosis), pathological data (e.g., incidence and prevalence of diseases), and to describe symptoms of diseases.

The ICD criteria for ADHD generally correspond with the DSM-IV-TR criteria but there are some distinctions in categorization and in the description of symptoms and in the diagnosis of ADHD. ADHD is referred to "Hyperkineticdisorder“ in the ICD and includes the following disorders:

1. Disturbance of activity and inattention
2. Hyperkinetic conduct disorder
3. Other hyperkinetic disorders
4. Hyperkinetic disorder, unspecified

Diagnostic criteria for ADHD in DSM-IV

Attention-Deficit/Hyperactive Disorder. Diagnostic criteria for ADHD in the DSM-IV.

A) Either(1)or (2):
   1) Six or more of the following symptoms of inattention have persisted for at least 6 months to a degree that is maladaptive and inconsistent with developmental level.

Inattention:

- often fails to give attention to details or makes careless mistakes in schoolwork, work, or other activities;
- often has difficulty sustaining attention in tasks or play activities;
- often does not seem to listen when spoken to directly;
- often does not follow on instructions and fails to finish schoolwork, chores, or duties in the workplace (not due to oppositional behavior or failure to understand instructions);
- often has difficulty organizing tasks and activities;
- often avoids, dislikes, or is reluctant to engage in tasks that require sustained mental effort (schoolwork or homework);

- often loses things necessary for tasks or activities (e.g., toys, school assignments, pencils, books, or tools);
- is often easily distracted by extraneous stimuli;
- is often forgetful in daily activities.
  2) Six or more of the following symptoms of hyperactivity-impulsivity have persisted for at least 6 months to a degree that is maladaptive and inconsistent with developmental level.

Hyperactivity:

- often fidgets with hands or feet or squirms in sea;
- often leaves seat in classroom or in other situations in which remaining seated is expected;
- often runs about or climbs excessively in situations in which it is inappropriate (in adolescents or adults, may be limited §8to subjective feelings of restlessness);
- is often "on the go" or acts as if "driven by a motor";
- often talks excessively.

Impulsivity:

- often blurts out answers before questions have been completed;
- often has difficulty awaiting turn;
- often interrupts or intrudes on others (e.g., butts into conversations or games)

B) Some hyperactive-impulsive or inattentive symptoms that caused impairment were present before age 7 years.
C) Some impairment from the symptoms is present in two or more settings (e.g., at school/work and at home).
D) There must be clear evidence of clinically significant impairment in social, academic, or occupational functioning.
E) The symptoms do not occur exclusively during the course of Pervasive Developmental Disorder, Schizophrenia, or other Psychotic Disorders and are not better accounted for by another mental disorder (e.g., Mood Disorder, Anxiety Disorder, Dissociative Disorder, or a Personality Disorder).

Criteria forHyperkinetic Disorder in ICD-10

F90 Hyperkinetic Disorder

Distinct inattention, over activity, and impulsivity must be present. These behavioral characteristics have been pervasive across all settings, have persistent, and are not better accounted for by other disorders, such as autisms or affective disorders.

Inattention

Six of the following symptoms have persisted for at least 6 months to a degree that is maladaptive and inconsistent with the developmental level of a child:

1) often fails to give close attention to detail or makes careless errors in schoolwork, work or other activities,
2) often fails to sustain attention in tasks or play activities,
3) often appears not to listen to what is being said to him or her,
4) often fails to follow through on instructions or to finish schoolwork, chores, or duties in the workplace (not because of oppositional behavior or failure to understand instructions),
5) is often impaired in organizing tasks and activities,
6) often avoids or strongly dislikes tasks, such as homework that require effort,
7) often loses things necessary for certain tasks or activities, such as school assignments, pencils, books, toys or tools,
8) is often easily distracted by external stimuli,
9) is often forgetful in the course of daily activities.

Overactivity

At least three of the following symptoms have persisted for at least 6 months to a degree that is maladaptive and inconsistent with the developmental level of a child:

1) often fidgets with hands or feet or squirm on seat,
2) leaves seat in classroom or in other situations in which remaining seated is expected,
3) often runs about or climbs excessively in situations in which it is inappropriate (in adolescents or adults only feelings of restlessness may be present),
4) is often unduly noisy in playing or has difficulty engaging quietly in leisure activities,

5) exhibits a persistent pattern of motor activity that is not substantially modifies by social context or demands.

Impulsivity

At least one of the following symptoms have persisted for at least 6 months to a degree that is maladaptive and inconsistent with the developmental level of a child:

1) often blurts out answers before questions have been completed,
2) often fails to wait in lines or await turns in games or group situations,
3) often interrupts or intrudes on others (e.g., butts into others' conversation or game),
4) often talks excessively without appropriate response to social constraints.

- Onset of the disorder has been present before age 7 and not beyond.
- Pervasiveness. Criteria must be met in more than one situation e.g., combination of inattention and over activity must be present at home and school, or elsewhere where the child is being observed e.g., at the clinic.
- Symptoms in 1-3 cause clinically significant impairment in social, academic, or occupational functioning.
- The disorder does not meet criteria for Pervasive Developmental Disorder (F84.-), Manic Episode (F30.-), Depressive Episode (F32.-), or Anxiety Disorders (F41.-).

(International Classification of Diseases, ICD-10)

1.3. Differential Diagnoses and Comorbidity of ADHD

1.3.1. Comorbid Diagnoses

Many symptoms of ADHD can be also observed in other diagnoses; therefore ADHD is comorbid with other psychiatric disorders. In many cases clinicians need to use a differential diagnosis in their assessment with their patients (e.g., if presented symptoms meet criteria for ADHD or for another diagnosis). If two or more disorders are present the first one should be considered as primary and the other secondary (e.g., persisting diagnosis of ADHD can lead to the development of secondary mood disorders or ADHD diagnosis exists concurrently with another psychiatric disorder).

Whether the diagnosis exists as primary or secondary it does not change the fact that ADHD is highly comorbid with other associated disorders. Up to 60 % of children with ADHD suffer from at least one comorbid disorder and many of these children have multiple diagnoses. [128, 86] Extensive epidemiological research of ADHD shows that 70 % of individuals with ADHD suffer from at least one additional disorder. [128] In analysis of the study, 40% of individuals with ADHD also suffered from ODD (Oppositional Defiant Disorder). Additionally, 14 % of children with ADHD also had CD (Conduct Disorder). Also, nearly 30 % of children with ADHD suffered from Anxiety Disorder, 10% had Tic Disorder, and 4 % had comorbid Mood Disorder. Findings in other studies show that 25-33 % of the individuals with ADHD have experience at least one depressive episode in their childhood. [34] United States statistics show almost one third of all children with ADHD suffer from learning disabilities. Another study on children with speech impairments found that children with ADHD are more likely to have impaired verbal communication. [29]

Common comorbid disorders with ADHD [86]

- Oppositional Defiant Disorder - as much as 50 %
- Conduct Disorders - 30 - 50 %
- Mood Disorders - 15 - 20 %
- Anxiety Disorders - 20 - 25 %
- Specific Learning Disabilities - 10 - 25 %

Other ADHD comorbid conditions are Tourette's syndrome, Recurrent somatic pain, Bipolar Affective Disorder, Mental retardation, Autism Spectrum Disorder, and Aspergers syndrome. [250] However, according to Dudova and Hrdlicka, Pervasive Developmental Disorder describes hyperactivity as *hyperactive behavior* as it relates to Hyperactive syndrome and not as a part of ADHD. Furthermore, there is insufficient evidence to prove children share characteristic of both disorders. [86]

Increased risk of substance abuse is expected to be higher in individuals with ADHD (e.g., alcohol, nicotine). Longitudinal studies found that individuals with a medical history of hyperactivity in their childhood are more likely to abuse alcohol and nicotine. [243, 205] Other findings show individuals with ADHD who did not receive proper treatment were more vulnerable to substance abuse in comparison to those individuals who received treatment for ADHD. [154] Additionally, smokers who were treated for ADHD stated they unintentionally smoked less in adulthood.

In another study, it was showed that more than 50 % of children with ADHD were observed to experience difficulty in applying social skills in acceptable manners when interacting with others. [186]

1.3.2. Differential Diagnoses

Differential diagnoses are disorders that can mimic ADHD in their symptomatology. These disorders can be misdiagnosed as ADHD and therefore need to be clearly differentiated from ADHD.

Decline in attention can be present in mental disorders, such as Mood Disorders and Anxiety Disorders, but can also be present in seizure disorder, head injuries, chronic physical diseases, in neglected and abused children, etc. [86] Autistic Spectrum Disorders and Mental Retardation are also usually connected with attention deficit and are considered the primary diagnoses.

Conduct Disorder without attention deficit is also difficult to distinguish from hyperactivity.

In 2002 Spencer et al. state some of the differences between ADHD and other disorders: [250]

- Individuals with *Conduct Disorders* differ from those with ADHD in persistent antisocial behavior, such as lying, deceiving, and robbery.
- Individuals with *Oppositional Defiant Disorder* are easily upset and exhibit hostile and negative behavior.
- Individuals with *Depressive Disorder* may exhibit problems with attention. However, criteria for the presence of depressive episodes must have duration of at least 2 weeks and involved decreased interest in activities and a loss of energy while still remaining hyperactive.
- *Bipolar Disorder* can in some cases be difficult to distinguish from ADHD. Individuals with Bipolar Disorder show obvious mood changes, euphoria, grandiosity, irritability, decreased need for sleep, etc.

- In the case of *Anxiety Disorders* hyperactive behavior is common. Symptoms include frequent fidgeting, inattention and accompanied by constant worry and fear.
- *Mental Retardation* unlike ADHD displays general intellectual disabilities and severe impairment in functioning in social settings, school and work.

Table 1. Overview of frequent ADHD comorbidities and their symptoms [86, 250]

Comorbidity	**Symptoms commonly shared by children with the following disorders**
Oppositional Defiant Disorder	temper tantrums, argumentative with adults, hostility towards authority figures, rule violations, aggressive and antisocial behavior, refusal to cooperate
Mood Disorders	sad mood, weeping, low self-esteem and insecurity as a result of failing school, difficulties forming relationships with peers, social isolation, and loss of interests
Anxiety Disorders	fear, anxiety, avoidance of certain situations, low self-esteem and insecurities as a result of failing school, difficulties forming relationships with peers, somatic symptoms
Learning disabilities	poor expressive language skills, sensorimotor coordination usually impaired, poor handwriting and ability to read does not match the expected developmental level for the chronological age of the child
Conduct Disorders	aggression towards others, destructive behavior, lying, stealing and robbery, rule violations
Tic Disorders	presence of motoric tics

- Individuals with *Developmental Disorders*, such as Autism Spectrum Disorder or Asperger syndrome may exhibit similar behavioral characteristics to individuals with ADHD. For Example, hyperactivity, inattention, impaired social functioning, and functioning at school or occupation. However, individuals with Developmental Disorders show additional symptoms, such as impairment in social interactions, presence of stereotyped behavior, stereotyped activities, similar interests, etc.

- *Learning Disorders* similar to ADHD also share similar characteristics and are often comorbid with ADHD. Individuals with Learning Disorders share difficulties with learning and significant differences in their academic work compared to their peers in relation to reading, writing, and math.

Table 1 shows the most common disorders that are comorbid with ADHD and the characteristics of these disorders that children possess.

1.4. Classification of ADHD

In the DSM-IV, a diagnosis of ADHD must be based on a complex assessment derived from interviewing various sources, such as the individual themselves, parents, and teachers. Also, the subject must undergo observation at home, school, and at the clinician's office. An additional psycho-diagnostic assessment of cognitive abilities must be administered (e.g., Conners Continuous Performance Test II CPT II) along with a behavioral rating scale (Conners - Parent, Teacher and Self-assessment). [63] In order to provide a reliable diagnosis, information about the individual with ADHD must be collected from **several individuals** whom interact with the subject, parents, teachers, therapists or other mental health care professionals along with and the individual them self. Furthermore, the information must be collected while **indifferent surroundings** (e.g., home, school), and other social settings (e.g., school activities, community centers). The above criteria help verify ADHD symptoms are persistent, pervasive, and maladaptive. The individual's behavior can vary throughout the school day depending on the individual's affinity for the educational topic. Assessments from the individual's teachers are also used to determine the diagnosis. Additionally, if an individual with ADHD lives within an environment of shared custody and in two different households, it is advisable to include the parent's observations of the individual. These assessment requirements are frequently beyond the scope of a routine clinical practice.

American Academy of Pediatrics developed clinical instructions to help in diagnosing and assessing children with ADHD. [5] These instructions include the Conners scale, which is a reliable instrument in identifying individuals with ADHD (CSR). [64]

1.5. Etiology of ADHD

The causes of ADHD are not fully understood today, but a number of factors exist that are believed to be contributing to the evolution of the disorder. In a sense, ADHD provides a model that illustrates the interaction among genetic, neurobiological, and epigenetic factors

Today, a greater importance is being places on the **genetic** components in ADHD. [20] The evidence from family studies showed that ADHD is often a multi-generational problem. The study also revealed that siblings of children with ADHD are also likely to suffer from ADHD. When twins are involved, the chance of being diagnosed with ADHD only increases which supports genetic factors playing a significant role in ADHD. It was further found that monozygotic twins have an 81% concordance rate - if one twin suffers from ADHD it is highly probable that the second twin will also suffer from ADHD. [106] A concordance rate of 29% was found in dizygotic twins. In general, studies involving ADHD symptoms in twins supported a heritability of 0.80. [256] Studies on adopted children also supported the heritability of the disorder. Findings of retrospective studies that focus on ADHD in parents whose children were diagnosed with ADHD showed that biological parents exhibited higher rates of hyperactivity than adoptive parents. Many researchers attempted to identify a specific gene responsible for ADHD and focused on identifying the dopaminergic genes (e.g., D2, DRD4, DAT1). Recent genetic studies show ADHD is mostly a polygenic disorder where several genes contribute to the disorder. [20]

In 2003 Kotimaa et al. together with other researchers indicate that etiology of ADHD may be associated with an exposure to **toxins** (in prenatal and postnatal period). [144] The medical history of children with ADHD often contains notes about mothers smoking and drinking alcohol during pregnancy. One of the prospective studies showed a correlation between a mother smoking during pregnancy and subsequent incidence of ADHD in her newborn baby. Therefore, the research indicated prenatal exposure to these substances may lead to ADHD. It was further found, that parents who suffer from ADHD drink and smoke more. Therefore, it is not clear that alcohol, nicotine, and the genetic component have a direct effect on ADHD. Epidemiological research also referred to the role of environmental toxins in ADHD, such as lead. [190] Some individuals with high levels of lead in the blood exhibited symptoms of ADHD but not all children with ADHD have high levels of lead in their blood. These findings suggest that lead poisoning may not be the primary cause of ADHD despite the fact that lead poisoning may be an important factor in the development of ADHD in some individuals.

The increased number of international adoptions from institutions raised awareness about the effect **neglect** has on children in their yearly development. Although many of these children (or children previously abused, tortured, or traumatized) show signs of inattention and overactivity their overall symptom manifestation qualitatively differs from the diagnosis in the DSM-IV-TR. The following study found that symptoms of inattention and overactivity associated with institutional environments are often accompanied with symptoms of Affective Disorder. [150]

Another potential cause of ADHD identified in the past was food allergies. [68] Some research projects further studied food consumption e.g., they focused on the relationship between fatty acids deficiency and ADHD. [241] This area of research continues to evolve, therefore no relationship between fatty acids and ADHD can be confirmed. [48]

The research on ADHD continues and the exact causes are not known with certainty. The following research findings were found to be consistent:

1) Most people suffering from ADHD have changes in brain anatomy and brain functioning;
2) ADHD has a genetic component or genetic risk factors that contribute to the development of the disorder;
3) Environmental factors play a role in ADHD manifestation;
4) Although not considered a primary cause of ADHD in all cases, prenatal exposure to toxins can explain some examples of ADHD.

1.6. Prevalence of ADHD

Some authors (e.g., Conners, Wells, Parker, Sitarenios, Diamond and Powell) state the prevalence of ADHD does not depend on age, gender, or socioeconomic status. Although, it can not be determined with certainty that the preceding factors do not play a role in ADHD. [64]

The previous conceptualization of ADHD presumed children with ADHD will eventually "outgrow" the disorder. However, today it is well known that many individuals continue to exhibit symptoms of ADHD through adolescence and adulthood. ADHD manifests itself differently at various stages of life and is expanded upon later in "Manifestations of ADHD across the lifespan". [268] Younger children mostly exhibit impaired inhibition in behavior and emotions. Some manifestations of ADHD change with age (e.g., motoric hyperactivity and impulsivity are viewed more as internal restlessness with difficulties becoming more apparent in social settings). [268]

Available research does not suggest ADHD is connected with race. ADHD also appears not to be associated with social class, though several studies identified lower prevalence of the disorder in ethnic minority groups. [88]

The literature offers extensive information about gender differences in ADHD and clearly shows higher prevalence in males than females. Only some longitudinal studies show the ratio of ADHD prevalence may be 1:1 between males and females. [15] Previous definitions of ADHD primarily focused on physical hyperactivity which resulted in more boys than girls being diagnosed with ADHD. Women and girls are more likely to exhibit symptoms of verbal hyperactivity (instead of the motoric symptoms), impulsivity, and possible weakening of executive functions, such as planning, emotional regulation, etc. Because the disorder impairs daily functioning in women less than in men, it is often not detected. The question of gender influence on ADHD is still unclear.

Additionally, ADHD can be diagnosed at any intellectual level provided symptoms of attention and self-control in children are inconsistent with the developmental level of the child (in case of mental retardation it is not necessarily the chronological age).

Manifestations of ADHD across the lifespan [268]

- *Infant age*
  - Individuals with ADHD already exhibit salient symptoms of the disorder as infants. The basic biorhythm is impaired (impaired sleep) and the child appears restless, irritable, often cries, and demands to be fed.
- *Toddler and preschool age*
  - At this stage the disorder manifests itself through impaired emotional and behavioral inhibitions. Children usually become excessively wild, react inadequately to situations, become upset, seek attention, run around, climb furniture, etc.
- *School age*
  - Problems arise when the child begins school and is required to conform to the rules of the school. School age children exhibit cognitive dysfunction, inattention, and lack of concentration that leads to poor academic performance (despite their good

intellectual ability). Children at this stage are irritable, sometimes act aggressively, and may suffer from a lower self-esteem.

- *Adolescence*
  - Adolescents with ADHD feel socially isolated and generally posses an impaired self-image. They tend to experiment with addictive substances and can exhibit behavioral problems.
- *Early adulthood*
  - Adults with ADHD may show social maladaptation. They are continually having difficulty organizing at work and school, have problems in relationships, and are in a risk category for substance abuse. Additionally, young adults tend to be subjected to the likelihood of engaging in illegal activities.

1.7. Summary

The evolutionary process of the terminology involved with ADHD has not been an easy path. Initially, the field focused on neurological factors but later moved towards describing the apparent behavior of the disorder. Currently, the most used name of the disorder is ADHD which comes from the English description "Attention Deficit Hyperactivity Disorder".

ADHD is currently one of the most used disorders to diagnose children. ADHD is a developmental disorder combining overactivity, impulsivity, and inattention. The disorder manifests itself as deficiency in the area of cognitive, executive, perception-motor skills, and social adaptation during the child's development. Up to 60 % children with ADHD also suffer from at least one comorbid disorder. The most frequent comorbid disorders are Defiant Oppositional Disorder, Conduct Disorders, Learning Disabilities, Mood Disorders, and Anxiety Disorder. The high comorbidity rate of ADHD complicates process of diagnosing, classifying, and treating the disorder.

The interaction of the genetic, neurobiological, and epigenetic factors contribute to the development of the ADHD model. Heritability and biological factors are considered the main causes of ADHD (e.g., abnormal fetal development, developmental impairment). Existing research shows dysfunctional genes in dopamine receptors, dopamine and serotonin transporter are responsible for the development of ADHD. Research has also showed environmental factors also play an important role in the development of ADHD.

Chapter 2

Biological Variability of ADHD

Abstract

The following chapter about biological variability of ADHD offers an overview of biological associations with ADHD, particularly neuroendocrine changes with a later chapter describing the genetic variability of ADHD. In individuals with ADHD specific characteristics are described in the brain neuroanatomy and in the neuroendocrine functions. Specific changes leading to chemical dysregulation in the brain contribute to the disorder. The chapter also discuss endocrine system functioning which may vary in patients with ADHD. Some authors talk about changes in the hypothalamic-pituitary-adrenocortical axis and stress hormone concentrations. The research also focused on changes in the endocrine functions in adipose tissue. Evidence of endocrine activity in ADHD brings important information to the clinician that helps provide abetter understanding of ADHD and its etiology.

2.1. Introduction

According to the majority of professionals and support from existing studies biological changes are seen as the major cause of ADHD. Based on these professional opinions and empirical findings, ADHD symptomatology is greatly influenced by dysfunction of certain brain areas. The dysfunction or changes in the brain are also likely genetically predetermined. Therefore, a great deal of research is focused on neuroanatomical and neurochemical changes. It is believed there are many changes in certain areas of the brain relating to volume (Emond, Joyal and Poissant), maturation (Shaw and Rabin) and activity (Clarke, Barry, McCarthy, Selikowitz, Clarke and Croft; Stark et al.). [90, 236, 59, 252]

Possible changes in the endocrine system that can play an important role in the symptomatology of ADHD are not given adequate attention. Further research on changes affecting symptomatology of ADHD also exists in the activity of stress hormones (Ma, Chen, Chen, Liu and Wang) and thyroid hormone levels (Stein and Weiss). [162, 253] Additionally, some studies of hormones found in adipose tissue show on a possible role in the development of ADHD. [220]

2.2. Neurobiology of ADHD

Empirical data show that specific changes at the brain level cause an alteration in the chemical regulation of the brain and are probably contributing to the development of ADHD. [77] These changes can be divided into neuroanatomical, neurochemical, and neurophysiological.

2.2.1. Neuroanatomical Changes

Imaging methods allow us to identify possible relationships between a brain morphology and psychiatric disorders. Computed tomography (CT) and magnetic resonance (MT, MRI) are also allowing analysis between the relationships of brain morphology and ADHD.

In 1999 Mostofsky, Wendlandt, Cutting, Denckla and Singer used imaging techniques to identify specific abnormalities of **frontal lobes**. [182] In his findings, Mostofsky described a lower density of gray matter in the right frontal lobe, even less gray matter in the left frontal lobe, and an overall smaller amount of white matter on both sides of the brain. The author indicates the right hemisphere is necessary for attention and that abnormalities in the structure and function of the right frontal lobe may contribute to behavioral deficiencies in ADHD. [182] These findings indicate children with ADHD have difficulties controlling their behavior because of their weakened ability to distinguish between relevant and irrelevant stimuli. Additionally, these findings contribute to the belief that ADHD is a disorder of "intention" (readiness to answer) which may be based in the differences found in the development of the frontal lobes.

The right hemisphere plays a key role in the development of social skills and this area appears to be problematic for individuals with ADHD. In 2006 Miller, Miller, Bloom, Hynd and Craggs found that children with ADHD who display morphological changes in their right hemisphere also experience significant difficulties with their social skills. [175] In 2002 Mala further states there is no apparent asymmetry in the hemispheres during fetal development. [164] However, the decrease of asymmetry of the right hemisphere is not isolated to ADHD but also can be found in disorders of early brain development.

Emond, Joyal and Poissant further confirmed and elaborated on the idea that the **front striatal** areas of the brain are responsible for the pathophysiology of ADHD. [90] They described reductions in overall brain volume, the prefrontal cortex, the basal ganglia, and the cerebellum. Similar findings were also introduced in 2002 by Castellanos et al. and other expert. [54, 146] Additional research Emond, Joyal and Poissant identified a significant reduction in size of the corpus callosum while other studies showed only parts of the corpus callosum decreased. [90, 161]

The key neuroanatomical characteristics of patients with ADHD can be summarized according to meta-analysis performed by Ellison-Wright, Ellison-Wright and Bullmore:

- There are volume changesin the **frontal lobe** and the **nucleus caudatus** in patients with ADHD.
- In the brains of patients with ADHD there is an overall **gray matter reduction** in the putamen and globus pallidus region.
- The **striatal** region plays an important role in the symptomatology of ADHD.
- Clinical studies of individuals with brain injuries found ADHD symptoms were associated with lesions in the right posterior **putamen** region. Reduction in these brain subregions are a result of injury or insufficient size and may lead to similar behavioral manifestation as those found in ADHD. [89]

In addition to changes in brain volume, another study shows some parts of the brain of children with ADHD have a probable **delay in cortical maturation**. In this case, the level of gray matter maturation in experiments showed a delayed of up to 3 years in comparison to the control group. [236,

238] The delay was most prominent in prefrontal regions that are important for control of cognitive processes including attention and "motor planning". [238, 237]

Anatomical brain changes in patients with ADHD are the focal point of clinical research and this research will surely make great strides in the effort to further understand ADHD. However, Ellison-Wright, Ellison-Wright, and Bullmore in 2008 emphasize that the problem with most research is the focus on brain regions that are easier to study (larger areas are easier to map and analyze than smaller areas with higher density), therefore these critical brain areas can be omitted. [89]

2.2.2. Neurophysiological Changes

The field of neurophysiology points to potential biological aspects as being the cause of ADHD. Better understanding of the biology enables clinicians to improve their to accurately diagnose and treat ADHD. To date, there is not a clear consensus of how electrophysiological correlates affect ADHD. Based on available research, children with ADHD show specific abnormalities that closely relate to the clinical manifestations of the disorder compared to children in the control groups.

A number of scientists believe ADHD occurs as a result of **chemical impairment** in the **prefrontal cortex** or in other areas associated with it. [255] Such impairment leads to disruption of inhibitors that drive appropriate emotional responses. As a result, individuals express an inadequate cognitive or behavioral response with decreased attention and control.

In his study, Sterman noted that more than 90 % of children with ADHD showed **changes in** their **EEG** patterns. [225] Particularly in the prefrontal and sensomotor cortex with reduced or inhibited activity in all cortical areas. It is important to mention that some of the changes are normal in children younger than 8 years, so it is important to carefully monitor the age groups through testing. In line with this finding Clarke, Barry, McCarthy, Selikowitz, Clarke and Croft in 2003 pointed out that children with the most prominent EEG abnormalities often appear more anxious and have a higher rate of behavioral impairment. [59] According to the neurophysiological view, these findings were interpreted as a manifestation of a low activation level in the CNS. This level is associated with reduced brain capacity during inhibition. Additionally, the most restless and inattentive children have a relatively reduced level of activation, a decreased ability to activate, and the limited ability to control their own activities.

Findings from functional magnetic resonance imaging (fMRI) show brain areas responsible for attention control, working memory, and inhibition response to be smaller and less active in individuals with ADHD. For example, in 1998 Paclt and Florian describes reduced blood flow and a reduced metabolic activity in the prefrontal and frontal limbic areas. [196] Bush et al. described anomalies in the anterior cortex activity and cognitive abilities in non-medicated individuals with ADHD. [49] The fMRI tests measured blood flow in the brain during a given task and it discovered individuals with ADHD had a longer reaction time and that different parts of the brain were activated compared to controls. The previous findings agree with Amen and Carmichael who found that 65 % children with ADHD have a blood flow that is significantly lower in their prefrontal cortex when completing tasks that require attention. [3] Additionally, in 1997 Amen and Carmichael found 22% of children with ADHD have a lower blood flow in the prefrontal cortex during a period of calm. [3]

Reduced activation in attention and cognition confirmed Silk, Vance, Rinehart, Bradshaw and Cunnington findings of hypofunction of the white brain matter in a group of 15 patients with ADHD between the ages of 8 and 18. [240] Using diffusion tensor imaging methods (DTI - Diffusion Tensor Imaging) researchers found developmental changes in the pathways of cortical white matter in the prefrontal areas and pathways surrounding basal ganglia and cerebellum. The findings reflect a possible decrease in the myelination of axons that can lead to a decrease in the speed of communication between neurons. [72] These findings may be important for diagnosis and treatment. [240]

In 2012 Cubillo, Halari, Smith, Taylor and Rubia reports that research points at structural and functional changes in the frontal cortical and frontal subcortical areas persist through adulthoodeven though the symptoms improve. [69] The analysis above indicates the existence of persistent functional changes in adults with ADHD. These changes relate to the dysfunction of cognition, attention, and motivation in the frontal-cortical and subcortical areas.

Limitations to the above research are found in a small sample of patients. Although individuals with ADHD exhibit certain differences in the brain functioning and its activity, it cannot be taken as gospel, as there is a level of variability in this area in the normal population. Criticism of the above studies and of the approach state that brain research is limited by small samples and thus cannot state with certainty if children with ADHD have typical and unique characteristics relating to size and activity of their brain. [77]

2.2.3. Neurotransmission Disorders

Brain studies on neurochemical processes refer to changes in dopamine and norepinephrine/noradrenaline neurotransmission occurring in the brain. [209, 226] The "catecholamine hypothesis" proposes that ADHD develops because of a decrease in catecholamine (dopamine and noradrenaline) in the brain.

Noradrenaline and dopamine are structurally similar neurotransmitters. Dopamine is the precursor to noradrenaline in the sympathetic nervous system, however, both neurotransmitters are relevant in the process of attention with each having a different role that complements the other. [156] Decreased dopamine activity in the frontal lobes leads to a decrease in cognitive functioning, such as memory, attention, and motivation. [226] Studies using animal models found that motoric hyperactivity is associated with hypo-dopaminergic (Cardinal, Pennicott, Sugathapala, Robbins and Everitt) and hyperdopaminergic states (Viggiano, Grammatikopoulos and Sadile). [52, 270] This provides evidence that both extremes are related to behavioral and cognitive dysregulation. [245]

Literature on this topic appears to present ambiguous and sometimes controversial information. In relation to ADHD, some studies showed increased dopamine levels while other studies showed decreased dopamine levels. [226] As indicated by Fusar-Poli, Rubia, Rossi, Sartori and Balottin in 2012 the dopamine level is closely associated with a long-term use of stimulants. [104] Published studies show the continued use of stimulants can cause the above mentioned ambiguities. Patients who never used stimulants show a decreased amount of dopamine transporters in the brain whereas patients who used stimulants for a long time showed anextremeincrease in the amount of dopamine transporters in the brain. This can be viewed as a compensatory mechanism in response to increased levels of dopamine where the body tries to build an amount of dopamine transporters.

2.3. Variability of Endocrine Activity in ADHD

In relation to a diagnosis of ADHD, there is certain literature that discuses neuroendocrine changes. Besides the dopaminergic and noradrenergic systems playing an important role in ADHD it is also believed dysregulation of the endocrine system and changes in the hormone levels are also. There is limited research to validate this theory and existing literature does not provide any definite answers to support the belief. Despite the lack of research and recorded data on this topicit is still considered relevant and should not be omitted.

2.3.1. Stress Hormones

According to experts, anomalies in the hypothalamic-pituitary-adrenocortical (HPA) axis activity have been, in some cases, associated with potential causative factors in psychopathology. [117] Existing research refers to the significance HPA axis has in ADHD. [162, 202, 46, 269]

The hypothalamic-pituitary-adrenocortical axis activity can be assessed through measuring the **cortisol** levels in the brain. Cortisol increases the overall readiness of an individual during stressful situations and has many effects, such as stimulation of the CNS where it increases stimulation and emotional instability. There are differences in the cortisol levels between children and adults as well as between genders. For example, a comparison of girls to boys shows that girls have higher basal activity resulting from stress. [117]

In 2010 Barzman, Patel, Sonnier and Strawn found higher cortisol levels occur in aggressive and impulsive individuals while lower cortisol levels were found in individuals who were lackingin emotion. [25] Stadler et al. in 2011 found lower cortisol levels may be associated with some disorders and were also described in children with ADHD. [251] Additionally, the level of the adrenocorticotropic hormone was also observed in the subject. However, the difference in the cortisol level between these individuals was not found. [162]

Table 2 presents an overview of findings about HPA axis activity. In some cases, a decreased basal cortisol level along with a decreased response to stressful stimuli was found which resulted in slow increase of the cortisol level. [138, 102, 162] This became evident in a group of children with ADHD who possessed hyperactive impulsive traits. It was noticed the children had significantly lower cortisol levels than children with either ADHD-predominantly inattention type or ADHD-combined type. Compared to controls the ADHD group (regardless of individual subtypes) had significantly lower cortisol levels (226.47±129.12 nmol/L ADHD vs. 384.53±141.43 nmol/L control group, P<0.001). [162] Differences in cortisol levels between individual subtypes were also described in 2009 by van West, Claes and Deboutte. [269] The study showed cortisol levels increased before and after exposure to stress in the ADHD-predominantly inattention type. On the other hand, in the ADHD-combined type (ADHD-C) cortisol levels were found to be significantly lower in comparison to the ADHD-predominantly inattentive type and in comparison to the controls. Additionally, van West, Claes and Debutte in 2009 reported decreased response levels were especially apparent in individuals with ADHD-C. [269]

The above research findings cannot be generalized because other studies could not find any significant difference in cortisol levels in ADHD patients. [116] Additionally, Freitag, Hänig, Palmason, Meyer, Wüst and Seitz in 2009 found only children with the comorbid disorder of Oppositional defiant disorder exhibited decreased cortisol levels while children with only ADHD and with ADHD and comorbid Conduct disorders and Anxiety disorders did not show deceased cortisol levels. [102]

Table 2. Hypothalamic-Pituitary-Adrenocortical Axis activity and ADHD [103]

Reference	Patient Population	Diagnosis/ Behavioral traits	Monitored Parameter	Results
Hatzinger, Brand, Perren, von Wyl, von Klitzing & Holsboer-Trachsler, 2007	102 (59 boys, 43 girls), age 5 years	Hyperactivity, impulsivity, emotional problems in boys, positive emotions in girls	Basal adrenal activity	Increased adrenal activity vs. controls
			Stress challenged adrenal activity	Increased adrenal activity vs. controls
Freitag, Hänig, Palmason, Meyer, Wüst & Seitz, 2009	128 ADHD, 6-13 years 96 controls, 6-12 years	ADHD with outcomorbidity and with comorbid ODD, conduct oranxiety disorders	Cortisol awakening response	Decreased cortisol in ADHD with comorbid ODD

Reference	Patient Population	Diagnosis/ Behavioral traits	Monitored Parameter	Results
	128 ADHD, 6-13 years	ADHD with current psychosocial riskor stress factors and ADHD without psycho social risk or stress factors		Increased cortisol with adverse family environment, family conflicts, and, acute life events
Hastings, Fortie, Utendale, Simard & Robaey, 2009	170 ADHD, school-age	ADHD with comorbid disruptive behavior and anxiety disorder, ADHD without these comorbidities	Salivary cortisol at waking, baseline	No differences in baseline cortisol levels in observed/monitored groups
			Salivary cortisol after stress exposure	Increased cortisol level after stress exposure in ADHD groups and with anxiety disorders
van West, Claes & Deboutte, 2009	76 ADHD, 6-12 years	ADHD-C, ADHD-I	Salivary cortisol during psychological testing of stress	In ADHD-I increased cortisol level compared to controls, in ADHD-C decreased cortisol level compared to controls
Barzman, Patel, Sonnier & Strawn, 2010	Children and adolescents	Impulsive and aggressive traits	Cortisol	Increased cortisol concentration
		Callous, without emotions		Decreased cortisol concentration
Stadler et al., 2011	36 boys with ADHD, 8-14 years	Higher callous, without emotions	Salivary cortisol before and after stress	Decreased HPPA activity in ADHD with higher callous compared to ADHD with a lower incidence of this feature
Ma, Chen, Chen, Liu & Wang, 2011	Boys with ADHD, 6-14 years	ADHD-HI, ADHD-I, ADHD combined type	Baselineat 8:00	Lowest cortisol level in ADHD-HI
			Level of adrenocorticotropic hormone (ACTH)	No difference
	boys, 6-14 years	ADHD vs. controls	Basal cortisol at 8:00	Lower baseline cortisol in ADHD
			Level of ACTH	No difference
Personen et al., 2011	272 ADHD, age 8 years	ADHD-IV Rating Scale and the Child Behavior Checklist (CBCL)	Diurnal salivary cortisol	No association between observed symptoms and diurnal cortisol level

Table 2. (Continued)

Reference	Patient Population	Diagnosis/ Behavioral traits	Monitored Parameter	Results
		ADHD-IV Rating Scale, CBCL, Trier Social Stress Test for Children (TSSTC)	Salivary cortisol after stress	Lower cortisol level after stress exposure in children with ADHD-I

Research monitoring changes in the activity of hypothalamic-pituitary-adrenocortical axis in individuals with ADHD is revealing inconsistent findings.

A lack of longitudinal studies in this area is the primary reason there is no clear interpretations of the findings from the research.

Variability in the findings results from the heterogeneity of subtypes in ADHD and from the incidence of comorbid diagnoses. [116] Other factors that contribute to the variability are; different methodsused to observe hormonal activity, the environmental influence on cortisol levels (stress events, family environment, school), and difficulties in ensuring consistent conditions in the test settings. [102]

Van West, Claes and Deboutte in 2009 reported other potential factors affecting research findings as stress events in the subject´s life and their experience with addiction. [269] They emphasize that ability to maintain the same conditions in test settings for every subject is not possible. Additionally, it cannot be determined if increased cortisol levels are the causing factors for problematic behavior or whether they are only accompanying features.

In regard to body growth, it must be noted that cortisol belonging to a group of glucocorticoids affects the production of the growth hormone. Glucocorticoids are generally known having an inhibiting effect on the growth hormone production.

Findings in children with ADHD who had lower cortisol levels could possibly contribute to diminished body growth as mentioned in professional publications. [213, 211] This is only a hypothesis and will be expanded upon later when the literature concerning this topic becomes publicly available.

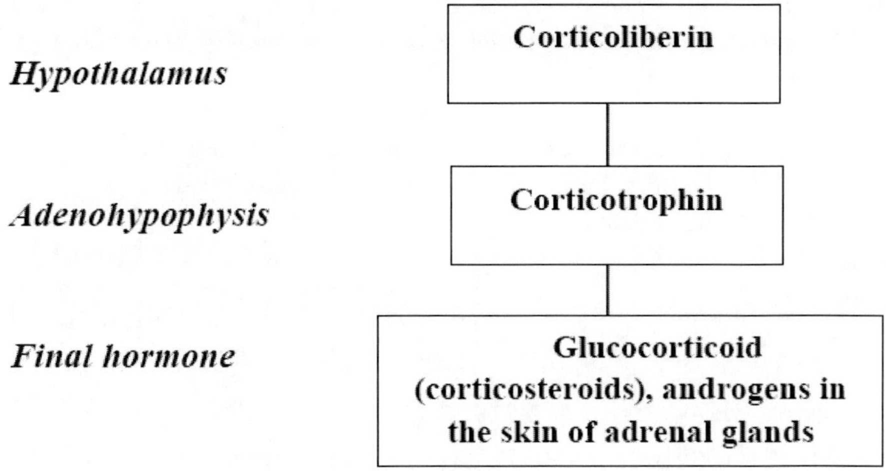

Figure 1. Effects of the corticotrophinaxis [242].

2.3.2. Thyroid Hormones

Thyroid hormone levels are another area of endocrine function being studied in patients with ADHD (triiodothyronine - T3, thyroxine - T4, thyrotrophin - TRH).

Thyroid hormone levels contribute to physical growth, especially during the prenatal period and during puberty. The hormone levels affect the metabolism of the entire organism. Future research could bring some very interesting findings about thyroid activity and how it relates to differences in physical development of individuals with ADHD. Unfortunately, these relationships have not been described in depth as of this date.

Published literature only provides evidence about changes in the thyroid activity in patients with ADHD and how the thyroid activity changes affect symptoms of hyperactivity and impulsivity.

Weiss, Stein, Trommer and Refetoff in 1993 reported prevalence of thyroid hormone abnormalities was higher in individuals with ADHD than in the normal population (5,4% vs. 1%). [278] This finding was later partially supported by Hauser, Soler, Brucker-Davis, Weintraub in 1997, who found a positive correlation between elevated thyroid hormone levels and symptoms of hyperactivity and impulsivity that match the DSM-IV criteria. [118] Thyrotropin did not correlate with symptoms hyperactivity and impulsivity. Triiodothyronine and thyroxineha a significant positive correlation with hyperactivity and impulsivity, but the levels of the hormones were not significantly correlated to inattention. Researchers further described a correlation between thyroid hormone concentration and symptoms of hyperactivity, however, the one does not cause the other. This research points at the importance thyroid hormones play in individuals with ADHD and also informs about the differences in an individual's functioning with symptoms of inattention and hyperactivity.

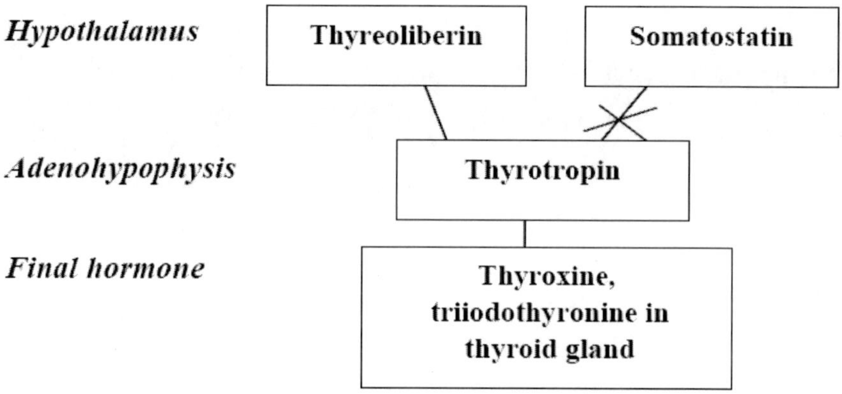

Figure 2. Effects of the thyrotrophicaxis [242].

Another research that identified differences in thyroid hormone levels in various ADHD types was done by Stein and Weiss in 2003. [253] Stein found low concentration of free toxins in the ADHD-predominant inattentive type but not in the ADHD-combined type. Concentrations of the free T4 were associated with individuals that exhibited mood liability, preoccupation, and lower ratings of attention. They were not associated with symptoms of hyperactivity which contradicts the findings of Hauser, Soler, Brucker-Davis and Weintraub in 1997. [118]

Significant differences in thyroid functioning were not found in studies by Spencer, Biederman, Wilens, Guite and Harding in 1995. [248] They observed moderate changes in thyroid hormone levels which were not statistically significant. Similarly, Toren et al. in 1997 found thattriiodothyronine levels were slightly above the norm for patients with ADHD, but there was not a significant difference between the individuals with ADHD and the control groups. [266] Additionally, Toren et al. found levels of total thyroxine, free thyroxine, and triiodothyronine showed normal levels.

Study results of thyroid functioning in individuals with ADHD, does not provide a comprehensive understanding of any correlation. Findings are contradictory and the majority are outdated and cannot be applied to clinical evaluations e.g., in diagnosis. [246]

2.3.3. Endocrine Function of Adipose Tissue

Patients with ADHD are often overweight or obese and studies on the endocrine function of adipose tissue explaining this relationship is limited.

Leptin, a hormone produced by adipocytes appears to have multiple functions in the body. It controls energy homeostasis, regulating the amount of fat and energy reserves stored in the body. Leptin also effects memory and the ability to learn. Leptin levels correlate with the BMI, the more adipose tissue there is, the more leptin there will be.

Reda and El-Hadidy in 2011 observed serum leptin levels in children and adolescents (age 6-18 years) with ADHD and who had a BMI value at or above the 95th percentile. [220] The level of leptin showed a positive correlation in relation to the BMI. They found a significant relationship between individuals with ADHD and controls when looking at IQ and the serum leptin levels. The levels showed a clear association with the IQ. Based on these findings, leptin could be an indicator of decreased cognitive function in individuals with ADHD. The relationship between leptin and appetite is well understood, but little is known about the relationship between the use of methylphenidates, which suppress the appetite, and leptin. [94] However, Iseri, Kilic, Senol and Karabacak in 2007 stated that short-acting methylphenidate in daily doses of 0.6 mg/kg neither influenced serum leptin levels nor lead to appetite suppression or changes in metabolism, as in the BMI and insulin and leptin levels. [126] Leptin levels can be associated with the dosage of methylphenidate as evidenced by animal studies that confirmed significantly higher leptin levels in case of a low dosage compared to levels at a higher dosage. [169] These findings may be important in clinical practice but they cannot provide any decisive conclusions about the relationship.

2.4. Summary

In individuals with ADHD, specific characteristics are described in the brain neuroanatomy and in the neuroendocrine functions.

Specific changes leading to chemical dysregulation in the brain contribute to the disorder. A series of changes in the brain were described, such as changes in the volume in some parts of the brain (Emond, Joyal and Poissant), the maturation (Shaw and Rabin) and the activity (Clarke, Barry, McCarthy, Selikowitz, Clarke and Croft; Stark et al.). [90, 236, 59, 252] Researchers were unanimous on their findings concerning the abnormalities in the structure and function of the right frontal lobe and its contribution to behavioral deficiencies associated with ADHD.

Endocrine system functioning may vary in patients with ADHD. Some authors talk about changes in the hypothalamic-pituitary-adrenocortical axis and stress hormone concentrations. They indicate decreased basal cortisol levels and cortisol levels after exposure to stressful situations. [251] Anomalies in functioning were also described in the thyroid gland and the production of its hormones; diiodothyronine and thyroxine. [253] The research also focused on changes in the endocrine functions in adipose tissue. Higher leptin levels in children with ADHD could be associated with either the decrease in cognitive functions or in changes in body weight. [220]

Evidence of endocrine activity in ADHD brings important information to the clinician that helps provide a better understanding of ADHD and its etiology. Additionally, these findings may lead to better clinical treatment and increase the effectiveness of that treatment and its planning.

Chapter 3

Genetic Variability in ADHD

Abstract

The following chapter presents an outline on how genetic factors play a role in ADHD. The proportion of genetic factors that contribute to the development of the disorder is about 75%. Family and twin studies on ADHD point at the high rate of heritability of the disorder. The most significant associations of genes are in the dopaminergic, serotoninergic, and noradrenergic systems. The genes with the most published association with ADHD are the DAT and DRD4 genes. There will also be discussion beyond the previously mentioned systems on how genes and their variants influence ADHD. Although the findings are very heterogeneous, ADHD is itself a heterogeneous disorder in its manifestation and genetic nature.

3.1. Introduction

Today's research shows ADHD to have a high rate of genetic origin. Studies from the late 1990's reported 30 - 35% of siblings of children with ADHD also meet the ADHD criteria. [33] Additionally, recent findings about monozygotic twins estimate heritability of ADHD to be near 75 %. [93] Genetic factors are certainly involved in the development of ADHD but the mechanism of how one obtains ADHD is not clearly understood. [70]

3.2. Genetic studies

Studies on families, twins, and adoption provide compelling evidence that genes play a strong role in the development of ADHD. Since families experience similar environmental factors, an emphasis is placed on twins and adoption studies. [131] A series of candidate genes that regulate the systems of neurotransmitters was described and a potential linkage between ADHD and specific chromosome regions was discovered on 5p13, 6q12, 16p13, 17p11, and 11q22-25. [98, 193] However, as of today most of the associations cannot be sufficiently proven. [100]

3.2.1. Family and Twin Studies

Adoption and twin studies show there is a strong genetic etiology for ADHD. [173, 194] In the late 1990's certain literature stated approximately 25% of adults with a history of hyperactivity have a child with ADHD. [33, 284] Additionally, existing literature references anaverage heritability rate of 76 %. [95]

There is also a strong relationship between heritability and comorbid disorders. Coolidge, Thede and Young in 2000 reported genetic etiology for ADHD, CD, ODD, and executive dysfunction. [65] They report heritability to be near 82% for ADHD, 74% for CD, 61% for ODD, and 77% for executive function.

3.2.2. "Linkage" Studies

A series of candidate genes is described in the case of heterogeneous disorders, one of which is ADHD. Linkage analysis is a robust method for identifying the presence of susceptibility genes for a genetic disorder. It is applied to a selected family group with a frequent incidence of disorder, or in a sample of siblings sharing a phenotype. The linkage analysis ultimately tests if the affected individuals share alleles more than by chance.

A limitation of the linkage analysis is the sample of tested individuals is too large. Fisher et al. in 2002 studied 126 twins and identified chromosomal regions at 2q24, 5p12, 10q26, 12p13, 12q23, and 16p. [98] A follow-up study of 270 twins identified significant linkage at 5p13, 6q14, 11q25, and 17p11. [193] Another linkage study of 308 children provided further evidence at

5p13, 6q12, and 17p11. [192] Bakker et al. in 2003 described evidence for locus on 5p13, 7p13 a 9q33 and Acosta, Arcos-Burgos and Muenke in 2004 found linkage at the 4q13, 5q33, 8q11, 11q22, 17p11, and at 8q11.23. [18, 1]

Based on the above results it is apparent the most replicated locus findings are 11q22 and 17p11. [1, 18, 98, 193] Recent studies confirmed genome-wide significance between 16q21-16q24. [1, 16, 18, 94, 119, 193, 224, 289, 288].

3.2.3. Association Studies

Association studies focus on testing relationships between specific allele, genotype or haplotype and the given disorder. They are used in the form of control studies and they compare the presence of the genetic variance between the experimental and control groups. Therefore, it is possible to test genetic variants of susceptible candidate genes or genes identified in the previous linkage analysis. Advances in technology are introducing better ways to include the use of association analysis in research today. For example, using methods of microarrays allows for a simultaneous testing of tens to hundreds of thousands single-nucleotide polymorphisms (SNP). [101, 100]

Attempts of genome-wide association studies were conducted to identify whole-genome linkage but these efforts did not produce any meaningful results. Franke, Neale and Faraone in 2009 stated the lack of results were a consequence of the sample sizes being too small to effectively unravel heterogeneity. [100]

A series of studied identified genes playing a role in the development of ADHD. However, this research lacks sufficient evidence to adequately demonstrate any specific genes directly cause ADHD. Despite the lack of evidence, it was discovered that potential candidate genes possibly exist that can contribute to ADHD. Some of the main candidate genes appear to belong to the dopaminergic, noradrenergic, serotoninergic, and GABAergic systems (genes for transporters and receptors of the transmitters as well as genes for enzymes, such as dopamine-β-hydroxylase, monoaminooxidase, and catechol-O-methyltransferase).

Molecular genetic studies focus mostly on genes in the dopamine system - dopamine receptor and dopamine transporter. Animal and humane studies point at the significance the dopamine system has in attention regulation. An existing relationship between ADHD and the dopamine system is supported by research that focuses on how stimulants block the reuptake transmitter and therefore increase the dopamine concentration in the synaptic cleft.

The most significant and most replicated candidate genes are the dopamine transporter gene (DAT), dopamine receptor gene (DRD1, DRD4, DRD5), and the monoaminooxidasa A gene (MAO-A). Current research is concentrating on the following genes: DRD4, DAT, DRD5, DBH, 5HTT, HTR1B, SNAP25, DRD2, DRD3, MAO, ADRA2A, GABA A3, and GABA B3. [93]

3.3. Genes and Their Variants

3.3.1. Dopamine System

DRD4 – The Dopamine Receptor Gene 4

Since the late 1990's, the dopamine receptor gene and how it affects postsynaptic dopamine activity has been the main focal point in association studies. DRD4 has highest rate of variability and is considered one of the most variable genes existing. Repetitive sequence (48 base-pair; bp) is important in coding the fourth cytoplasmic loop which is responsible for building the guanine-nucleotide proteins. Reporting from research on DRD4 and ADHD shows a frequent incidence of the 7-repeat allele in the sequence of variable tandem repeats in the coding sequence of the gene. This allele was found in 41% ADHD patients compared to 21% in the controls. Association studies of this repetitive allele and ADHD, is one of the most replicated and published studies on genetic variants in ADHD. [115]

DAT1 – The Dopamine Transporter Gene

The dopamine transporter gene DAT1 (*SLC6A3*) is another candidate gene that participates in dopaminergic transmission. Research repeatedly confirmed that association exist between ADHD and the presence of the 10 variable tandem repeats (VNTR) (480 bp) within the 3´-Untranslated region of DAT1. [130] It was found that individuals with a 10-repeat allele have approximately a 50 % increased density in this region compared to other individuals with different genotypes. This finding aligns with the results of imaging studies that identifies an increased density of dopamine transporters in the striatum. [130]

A number of authors also discuss the importance of variants 7-R DRD4 and 10-R DAT1. [229] The 7-R allele DRD4 may produce a receptor which is subsensitive to dopamine whereas allele 10-R of the gene DAT1 may be associated with high effect of dopamine re-uptake. Purper-Ouakil, Wohl,

Mouren, Verpillat, Ades and Gorwood in 2005 compared family-based association studies with a focus on gene variants DAT1 a DRD4. [216] They found that DAT1 plays a minor role in ADHD but in general the associations of these genes with ADHD are not significant. While studies focus more on the 10-R allele DAT1, some specific linkages with other mutation directly influence the DAT1 protein function. Additionally, environmental factors may also play a role in the process.

Durston et al. in 2005 stated that DAT1 is expressed predominantly in the basal ganglia, preferentially in the caudate whereas DRD4 is expressed predominantly in the prefrontal cortex. [87] They demonstrated the usefulness of combining molecular genetic studies with imaging methods which helped identify gene expression in brain regions which are important in the process of attention.

DRD1 – The Dopamine Receptor Gene D1

The DRD1 gene encodes the dopamine receptor gene D1 which is the most prevalent dopamine receptor in the CNS. DRD1 controls neuronal growth and differentiation while also allowing for behavioral responses. Genetic analysis identified different polymorphisms inside this gene and specifically identified the polymorphism A-48G DdeI as being mostly associated with ADHD. [40]

DRD2 – The Dopamine Receptor Gene D2

The DRD2 gene encodes the dopamine receptor gene D2 and is the most studied gene in psychiatry, especially in individuals with alcohol and nicotine dependency. The A1 allele (polymorphism TaqIA) is associated with the decreased expression of the gene and therefore is associated with decreased receptor density D2 in the striatum. [152] Amidst all these studies the association with ADHD was not clearly proven. Some authors, for example Paclt, Drtilkova, Kopeckova, Theiner, Sery and Cermakova in 2010 reported a strong positive correlation between the combined type ADHD and ANKK1 while meta-analysis done by Gizer, Ficks and Waldman in 2009 did not include this variant among the risk factors for ADHD. [197, 107]

DRD3 – The Dopamine Receptor Gene D3

The DRD3 is a gene for the D3 receptor and is located in the limbic areas of the brain and is associated with cognitive, emotional, and endocrine functions. The variants Ser9/Gly exhibit differential affinity for dopamine and thus the gene DRD3 is suspected of having a possible association with ADHD.

[185, 143, 75] Gene DRD3 is also at the center of pharmacogenetic research on treatment efficacy in ADHD. These more recent findings are countered by Muglia, Jain and Kennedy in 2002 whose research showed DRD3 plays an insignificant role in ADHD. [185]

DRD5 - The Dopamine Receptor Gene D5

The DRD5 is a gene for the D5 receptor and its (CA)(n) polymorphism is together with the other genes of the dopaminergic system associated with ADHD. Although studies again show significant heterogeneity, meta-analysis shows that the 148 bp allele is significantly associated with ADHD. [107]

DBH –The Dopamine-beta Hydroxylase Gene

The DBH gene is responsible for synthesis of the enzymes in dopamine-beta-hydroxylase and the gene catalyzes the oxidative hydroxylation of dopamine to noradrenaline [180] The DBH gene is also one of the candidate genes for Anxiety Disorders (Itoi and Sugimoto) and ADHD (Paclt, Koudelova, Pacltova and Kopeckova). [127, 198]

The variant DBH-1021C/T is associated with decreased dopamine-beta-hydroxylase activity, Disruptive behavior disorder, and ADHD. [287] Zhang, Du, Zhuang and Liu in 2005 reported the T allele is associated with ADHD-combined type especially in cases where ADHD exists together with behavioral comorbid disorders. [287]

A significant association of ADHD exists with other SNP especially with rs2519152 polymorphism. [74, 30] Polymorphisms rs2519152, rs1611115, and rs1108580 closely correlate with the dopamine-beta-hydroxylase activity. Meta-analysis of six studies, with significant heterogeneity across studies confirmed a relationship between two functional polymorphisms (rs1108580 and rs1611115) and low DBH concentration in the plasma. [107]

3.3.2. Serotoninergic System

SLC6A4 – The Serotonin Transporter Gene (5HTT)

This gene encodes the serotonin transporter and its long polymorphisms in the premotor region. This gene is among the most studied genes associated with several psychiatric disorders. The short variation (S) is associated with a lower transporter activity, a higher sensitivity towards stimuli that evoke anxiety and fear, and a higher rate of depressiveness and anxiety. [39] Allele L is more likely to contribute to manifestations of aggression, psychomotor unrest, and mood liability. However, literature describes controversy regarding the association of the serotonin transporter gene and ADHD. [151] Additionally, literature states that the S/S genotype exist with a lower frequency in individuals with ADHD compared to individuals in the normal population. ADHD individuals are more frequent heterozygous and homozygous L/L. However, some authors point at the association of the L/L genotype and how it manifests in elevated aggression, psychomotor unrest, and mood lability. [151]

HTR1B – The Serotonin 1B Receptor Gene

Certain studies show an association between the 1B serotonin receptor and ADHD. [218, 244] Meta-analysis of nine studies showed a moderate but significant effect of the 861G allele. [107] The authors found an association between the 5HT1B receptor gene and the inattentive subtype of ADHD. [244]

3.3.3. Noradrenergic System

ADRA 1A - Gene for Adrenergic α 1A-receptor

The noradrenaline system influences attention, ability to learn, and memory. ADRA 1A is significant in ADHD pathogenesis because of the knowledge about medication effects (methylphenidate increases catecholamine activity by increasing alpha 2A activity of the adrenergic receptors) and from the knowledge from animal studies. [13]

In ADRA 1A the GG genotype was observed in polymorphism 1291C-G SNP (rs1800544). Although Roman, Polanczyk, Zeni, Genro, Rohde and Hutz in 2006 and Roman, Schmitz, Polanczyk, Eizirik, Rohde and Hutz in 2003 described an association of ADRA 1A with the ADHD-inattentive and the ADHD-combined type, however, meta-analysis of 11 studies did not confirm this relationship (Gizer, Ficks and Waldman). [221, 222, 107]

ADRA 2A – Genefor Adrenergic α 2A-receptor

Similarly, research focuses on the relationship between the ADRA 2A gene and its one-nucleotide polymorphism in the premotorregion A-1291 C>G. The polymorphism of the gene creates a space for the restriction enzyme *MspI*. Thepolymorphism is associated with ADHD and shows the noradrenergic system plays an important role in ADHD etiology. [232]

SLC6A2 – Gene for the Noradrenaline Transporter

The gene for noradrenaline transporter is expressed in the frontal cortex and regulates reuptake of noradrenaline and dopamine. Although the noradrenaline system is considered to be significantly associated with ADHD, the association with polymorphisms in the gene of this transporter was not clearly identified (SNP rs5569 in exon 9 and SNP T - C in intron 13 - rs2242447). [107]

3.3.4. Other Genes

COMT - Gene for Catechol-O-methyl Transferase

Catechol-O-methyl transferase is an important enzyme in the process of catecholamine degradation (dopamine, epinephrine, and norepinephrine). The one-nucleotide variant (SNP) Val158Met in this gene causes dopamine catabolism to occur four times faster and therefore causes reduction in the dopaminergic stimulation of the postsynaptic neuron. Heinz and Smolka in 2006 report, that although this variant greatly influences the enzymes activity, it only has a moderate effect on behavior. [120] However, the variant influences working memory, executive function, and attention. The association between the enzymes activity and ADHD was confirmed by some researchers (Nobile et al.; Heinz and Smolka) while other researchers found the association was not completely clear (Mills et al.) [191, 120, 178]

SNAP 25 – Synaptosomal - Associated Protein

SNAP25 is a neuron-specific protein which contributes to catecholamine release. This gene is also considered another candidate for ADHD. [145] Studies have found an association of the two SNP variants (T1069C and T1065G) with ADHD. [43, 137]

TACR1 – Gene for Tachykinin Receptor 1

The gene for the tachykinin receptor is located in the prefrontal cortex and has not received much attention through studies. Although, studies on animal models found that the removal of this gene does leads to hyperactivity. [281] During tests mice exhibited decreased dopamine concentration in the prefrontal cortex and a diminished response to amphetamine. Yan et al. in 2010 reported a combination of certain neurochemical abnormalities in mice, together with their atypical response to psychostimulants that mimicked the characteristics of ADHD. [281] They further pointed at a relationship between TACR1 gene and affective subtype of ADHD.

TPH1 a TPH2 – Genefortryptophan Hydroxylase 1 and Genefor Tryptophan Hydroxylase 2

Tryptophan hydroxylase (TPH) controls the speed of neurotransmitter serotonin synthesis. Both forms of TPH1 (expressed in a series of peripheral tissues) together with TPH 2 (expressed in neurons) are considered ADHD related. Patients with ADHD were identified with polymorphism in intron 7 (rs1800532) (Li et al.) and this association was further confirmed by meta-analysis (Gizer, Ficks and Waldman). [158, 107] The previously mentioned meta-analysis did not confirm the significance of TPH 2 and the T allele (rs1843809) in ADHD. However, a certain portion of the studies did show the significance of the gene in the pathogenesis of ADHD. [274, 239]

MAO - Monoamine Oxidase

Monoamine oxidase A and B catalyze the deamination of monoamines, dopamine, noradrenaline, and serotonin. In the 1980's research found MAO inhibitors improve symptoms of ADHD which brought increased attention to studies involving monoamine oxidase as it relates to ADHD. [285] Other studies found functional polymorphism VNTR that consist of 2 to 3 copies is associated with impulsivity and aggression (Manuck, Flory, Ferrell, Mann and Muldoon) and that polymorphisms for this gene relate to ADHD (Jiang et al.). [166, 129] On the other hand, Gizer, Ficks and Waldman in 2009 in their meta-analysis did not find these results to be significant. [107]

3.4. Summary

The last decades have been characterized by intensive research on candidate genes and their significance in psychiatry, but the methodology used in these studies are not consistent and can cause inconsistent results. The inconsistent results may be caused by many factors - small number of samples, heterogeneity of monitored diseases, significant ethnic and national diversity of studies, and differences in distribution of the mentioned polymorphism. Of particular importance was the differentiation in the distribution of alleles in the population that made it difficult to interpret, compare, and generalize results.

Research on genetic variants that contribute to ADHD is considered to be current. The proportion of genetic factors that contribute to the development of the disorder is about 75%. Family and twin studies on ADHD point at the high rate of heritability of the disorder. Clinical genetic studies are concerned with genes in the dopaminergic, serotonergic, and noradrenergic systems and also stress the importance of areas 5p and 17q. The genes with the most published association with ADHD are the DAT and DRD4 genes. Although the findings are very heterogeneous, ADHD is itself a heterogeneous disorder in its manifestation and genetic nature.

There are many promising associations found in researching candidate genes and their variants, but the extent of our knowledge today is more theoretical than factual. To better understand the disorder we must further study the genetic factors, the heterogeneity of symptoms, and the incidence of comorbidity. The variability in the response to the treatment of ADHD is highly likely caused by genetic factors which were the main subject of the research in the first pharmacogenetic studies on ADHD. Pharmacogenetics in ADHD is still in the early stages and further research is needed before the findings can be used in the clinical practice. [210]

Chapter 4

Variability of Physical Growth in ADHD

ABSTRACT

This chapter discusses variability of physical development in children with ADHD. It introduces study results from research that monitored physical development in individuals with the disorder, results observing changes in physical development of medicated children and how it associates with the use of medication. According to several studies children with ADHD can achieve lower physical growth rates while having higher BMI values and a greater proportion of fat in their adipose tissue. The chapter provides a summary of studies on growth in ADHD children and studies on the effects of stimulant use on growth and development. Despite the attention received, the causes and associations between ADHD and growth are still not clear.

4.1. Introduction

Children with ADHD have been observed to experience changes in their mental and physical development. [211-214] Existing research shows these changes are especially illustrated in height, weight, and in fat deposits in the body tissue (Ptacek, Kuzelova and Paclt; Ptacek, Kuzelova, Paclt, Zukov and Fischer), and through an increased incidence of obesity (Bazar, Yun, Lee, Daniel and Doux; Waring and Lapane). [211, 214, 26, 275]

Changes in growth and weight are often attributed to the side effects of stimulant use, which are the most common psychopharmacological drugs. [79] The stimulant treatment may be accompanied by side effects, such as growth suppression, decreased appetite, and weight loss. [24] Current studies show that changes in body growth are probably associated with the disorder and that the stimulant treatment is not the primary cause. [214]

4.2. Physical Development and Its Changes in Children with ADHD

ADHD is associated with numerous biological changes and is believed to be associated with some specific changes in the body growth. These changes were studied together with the use of medication for an extended period and the side effects from the stimulant use (especially methylphenidate), such as growth suppression and decreased appetite were reported. In his study Poulton in 2005 found the use of methylphenidates caused weight loss on average of 1kg/year and delay in growth of 1cm/year. [206]

Although multiple studies exist on the effects of stimulant use has on child growth, there are few studies that focus on growth changes in children with ADHD.

One of the first studies on stimulants and child growth was done by McGee, Birkbeck and SIlva in 1985. [170] They measured basic physical parameters and skeletal maturity in a group of seven years old boys. They were expecting delayed physical development because of the delay in skeletal maturity however, this hypothesis was not confirmed. Swanson, Sergeant, Taylor, Sonuga-Barke, Jensen and Cantwell in 1998 analyzed findings from several studies and found that height in children treated with stimulants does not differ from the norm. [263] The average height in children with ADHD was reported to be in the 51st percentile and weight was in the 61st percentile. Additional data showed children treated with stimulants were found to be smaller than children in the controls.

A series of studies were done on height and body mass index (BMI) in children with ADHD. Altafas in 2002 pointed out that ADHD children are more prone to obesity. [2] In his study he found that individuals with ADHD who were in a weight loss program lost weight on an average 2,6 BMI (kg/m2) whereas individuals in the same group without ADHD lost an average weight of 4 BMI (kg/m2). [2] The difference in weight loss in individuals with an initial BMI higher than 40 was even more pronounced. Individuals with ADHD lost 2,9 BMI (kg/m2) and individuals without ADHD lost almost 7 BMI (kg/m2). Altafas explains in his findings that the characteristics of ADHD are what causes that individuals with ADHD are not so successful with weight reduction. [2] The incidence of a higher percentage of obese individuals who were unsuccessful at losing weight may be explained by the simple fact that they are may be explained be the simple fact that they are less persistent in efforts to achieve weight reduction. It was later described that obese individuals with attention or conduct disorders have greater difficulties losing weight. [71] Altafas stated also dopamine and insulin receptor activity may play a role in that process. [2]

Table 3. Comparison of studies observing growth parameters in children with ADHD

Reference	Average age for the observed groups (in years)	Observed parameters	Results
McGee, Birkbeck & Silva, 1985	7	BMI, height, weight, skeletal maturity, peripheral dimensions, triceps andsubscapular fat-folds	Statistically insignificant
Holtkamp et al., 2004	5,5 - 14,5	BMI	Higher BMI
Mustillo, Worthman, Erkanli, Keller, Angold & Costello, 2003	9-16	BMI	Not statistically significant
Curtin, Bandini, Perrin, Tybor & Must, 2005	3–18	BMI	Not statistically significant
Lam & Yang, 2007	13-17	BMI	Higher BMI, but not significant
Swanson, Sergeant, Taylor, Sonuga-Barke, Jensen & Cantwell, 1998	6-17	Height, weight	Higher values of height and weight
Waring & Lapane, 2008	5-17	BMI	Higher BMI
Hubel, Jass, Marcus & Laessle, 2006	8-14	BMI, basal metabolism BMR	Higher BMI, BMR
Ptacek, Kuzelova, Paclt, Zukov & Fischer, 2009a	6-12	Height, weight, BMI, peripheral dimensions, skinfold	Higher value of weight and proportion of fat deposits in the body tissue

Research focuses on obesity prevalence and the identification of risk groups, especially in the United States, who are predisposed to obesity. Several studies reported a relation between obesity and psychiatric diagnoses. [275] Similarly, Mustillo, Worthman, Erkanli, Keller, Angold and Costello in 2003 also found individuals with obesity exhibit a higher prevalence of psychopathology, especially conduct and attention disorders. [188] In the past it was assumed individuals with ADHD who show increased activity will exhibit a lower prevalence of being overweight and obese. [121]. But other studies proved otherwise as they found higher BMI values and percentage of body fat (Holtkamp et al.; Hubel, Jass, Marcus and Laessle; Waring and Lapane; Ptacek, Kuzelova, Paclt, Zukov and Fischer; Ptacek, Kuzelova and Paclt) in children as well as in adolescents (Lam and Yang) [121, 124, 275, 213, 211, 153]). In some cases higher BMI values did not reach a significant level, as was evidenced by the experimental group. [153, 188]

Hubel, Jass, Marcus and Laessle in 2006 supposed that obesity in individuals with ADHD is caused by impulsive behavior and therefore to some impulsive behavior in food consumption. [124] Different hypothesis about eating habits in children with ADHD are the subject of much research today.

Table 3 presents an overview of studies on physical changes in children with ADHD.

4.3. Physical Growth and Its Changes in Medicated Children with ADHD

Most research on physical growth in ADHD is aimed to study associations with pharmacotherapy. The first findings on body weight during treatment using methylphenidate and dextroamphetamine combined with a reduction in growth rate were published already in the 1970's. [228, 227] Many authors proved that at the beginning of treatment individuals with ADHD exhibited growth deceleration. [79]

Information is found in literature that weight loss, growth deficit, and reduction in growth velocity at the beginning of the treatment continues up to three years. [79, 208] However, most longitudinal studies do not last longer than three years and it is difficult to evaluate a long term effect medication may have had on the previously mentioned growth changes.

4.3.1. Cross-Sectional Studies

One of the first cross-sectional studies appeared in the early 1970's. They studied 'drug holidays' in 29 children and found that children without continuous treatment with stimulant medication exhibited double of growth rate compared to the group that was consistently medicated. [228]

Spencer, Biederman and Wilens in 1998 also studied growth changes. [247] They studied children who received treatment and found that younger participants had a more apparent growth delay that was in the range of1-3 cm - 2 SD from the mean. Similar changes in growth reported also the MTA Cooperative Group in 2004 and Charach, Figueroa, Chen, Ickowicz and Schachar in 2006. [184, 55]

Swanson et al. in 2006 described growth deficit and weight loss in the experimental group. [262] Differences between the experimental and the control group were on an average 2 cm and 2.7 kg – lower values were recorded by the group that received medication. Lisska and Rivkees in 2003 also reported similar findings between twins (with or without treatment) after two years of observation. [160] Finding of lower growth rates did not correlate with the dose amount of methylphenidate (10-80 mg/day) but was linked to a delay in growth. The authors of this study believe the dosage of medication does not play any significant role in growth changes. Other authors however, consider the dosage to have a significant influence on physical development. [235, 94] Based on these findings it is apparent more factors are contributing to physical changes. According to Schertz, Adesman, Alfieri and Bienkowski in 1996 a significant predictor of weight loss after the treatment began was the subject's weight prior to treatment. [231] According to researchers the weight prior to the treatment will determine if there will be any significant changes or no changes in the subject's weight during treatment.

However, cross-sectional studies have so far not produced any consistent findings. For example, Sund and Zeiner in 2002 did not confirm there is a relationship between treatment and growth in groups treated with methylphenidate and amphetamine. [260] Based on their findings treatment did not have any negative effects on growth. Also, similar conclusions were reached by Spencer, Faraone, Biederman, Lerner, Cooper and Zimmerman in 2006, Pliszka, Matthews, Braslow and Watson in 2006, Faraone and Giefer in 2007, and Ptacek, Kuzelova Paclt, Zukov and Fischer in 2009, Ptacek, Kuzelova and Paclt in 2009, Rose, Reeves, Gut and Germak in 2011 [249, 203, 92, 2013, 211, 225]

Other research provided unconvincing results when studying atomoxetine and changes in body growth Spencer, Faraone, Biederman, Lerner, Cooper & Zimmerman in 2006. [249] Data from experiments showing a decrease in height and weight rate were also published and this data also provided unpersuasive results. [147, 149]

4.3.2. Longitudinal Studies

Longitudinal studies are educating us about associations of treatment and long term changes in physical development. Although some experts tried to gain information about the mentioned association from retrospective studies while observing adult patients (Spencer, Biederman and Wilens) only longitudinal studies allow for the accurate description of changes over time. [247]

Zhang, Du, Zhuang and Liu in 2005 described height velocity in children treated with methylphenidate (0,27-0,64 mg/(kg)). [287] In his study, Zhang reports a gradual deceleration of height velocity in association with the duration of treatment (1st year 4,28 cm/year, 2nd year 4,90 cm/year, 3rd year 4,98 cm/year, 4th year 4,95 cm/year). Differences in weight were not found.

Faraone and Giefer in 2007 observed children from 6-12 years during a 3 year period of treatment with methylphenidate. [92] The results showed small but significant delays in growth and lower values for BMI and weight. Similar findings were also confirmed by Faraone, Biederman, Morley & Spencer in 2008 who added the effects of long term stimulant use depends on the dosage level and not on the specific drug (methylphenidate or amphetamine). [94] Although these changes occur over time they are so minute and do not have any on effect on height in adulthood. [94]

This was also confirmed by Zachor, Roberts, Hodgens, Isaacs and Merrick in 2006 whose results showed height in adulthood is the same in the experimental as well as the control group. [283] The results showed that any initial growth deficit at the beginning of the treatment did not have any long term effect on the ultimate height of the individual. They observed 89 patients during a 3 year period and evaluated the physical development in the intervals of the 3rd, 6th, 12th, 24th, and 36th months. During the first few months they found a significant weight loss in patients. Pre-pubertal children had a greater tendency to lose weight but after 2 years of treatment any significant changes were no longer apparent.

In the last few years experts are leaning towards the opinion that medication does not have any significant effect on physical development. One of the latest longitudinal studies analyzed children of both genders (age 8.6 + 1.7 years) who were treated with methylphenidate (dosage 0,41-0,49 mg/kg/day). Their study did not prove that treatment had any significant effect on physical development. Children were measured after 6 months of treatment and then every year for the next five years. After 6 months of treatment they observed the height in the subjects was lower ($p < 0.05$) and any other variables ere no longer considered significant. [183] Biederman, Spencer, Monuteaux and Faraone in 2010 carried out long-term studies for ten years in which they observed 124 individuals of both genders who were treated by some kind of stimulant and were compared to controls. [37] However, they also could not prove that stimulant use has an effect on height and weight. Although most of the research was done on boys, because of the ADHD prevalence in boys, it was discovered there were no differences in ADHD-growth association with treatment between boys and girls. [35]

The following table is an overview of findings of physical changes in association with medication. Evidence shows a deceleration in growth and weight loss in some cases. This is apparent in methylphenidate treatment, amphetamine treatment, and atomoxetine treatment. Unfortunately, the study results are not definite and in some cases there was no apparent statistical significance. The differences in the findings may be explained by such factors as heterogeneous methodology, dosage, relatively broad age span, short duration of studies, and very limited selection of observed parameters. Also, any observed body changes due to medication use appeared not to be statistically significant.

Table 4. Comparison of studies on the effects of medication on physical parameters

Reference	Age (in years)	Dose (mg/day)	Results
Safer, Allen & Barr, 1972	NS	mph ±20 mg (+ dex)	weight loss
Safer & Allen, 1973	NS	mph ±20 mg (+ dex)	growth suppression
Millichap & Millichap, 1975; Millichap, 1978	NS	mph 10-20 mg	no significant differences

Table 4. (Continued)

Reference	Age (in years)	Dose (mg/day)	Results
Kalachnik, Sprague, Sleator, Cohen & Ullmann, 1982	5-10	mph 18,4 mg	no significant differences
Klein, Landa, Mattes & Klein, 1988	6-15	mph < 60 mg	no significant differences
Vincent, Varley & Leger, 1990	12-18	mph = NS	no significant differences
Schertz, Adesman, Alfieri & Bienkowski, 1996	NS	mph = NS, dex = NS	weight loss
Spencer, Biederman & Wilens, 1998	12-18	mph24-38 mg	growth suppression
Swanson, Sergeant, Taylor, Sonuga-Barke, Jensen & Cantwell, 1998	6-17	mph 14,2 mg	growth suppression
Spencer, Biederman & Wilens, 1998	13-17	mph 19,8 mg	growth suppression
Sund & Zeiner, 2002	3-10	mph 23,9 mg; dex 11,9 mg	no significant differences
Biederman, Faraone, Monuteaux, Plunkett, Gifford & Spencer, 2003a	6-17	mph = NS	no significant differences
Lisska & Rivkees, 2003	NS	mph 10-80 mg	growth suppression
Poulton & Cowell, 2003	6-18	mph 27 mg; dex 13,7 mg	growth suppression
MTA cooperative group, 2004	NS	mph 34,4 mg	growth suppression

Reference	Age (in years)	Dose (mg/day)	Results
Zhang, Du, Zhuang & Liu, 2005	NS	mph 27-64 mg	growth suppression
Spencer, Faraone, Biederman, Lerner, Cooper & Zimmerman, 2006	4-12	amx 1,8 mg	no significant difference
Charach, Figueroa, Chen, Ickowicz & Schachar, 2006	6-12	mph = NS	weight loss
Zachor, Roberts, Hodgens, Isaacs & Merrick, 2006	NS	mph = NS	weight loss
Kratochvil et al., 2006	6 -7	amx = NS	growth suppression, weight loss
Pliszka, Matthews, Braslow & Watson, 2006	NS	mph = NS; dex = NS	no significant differences
Faraone & Giefer, 2007	6-12	mph = NS	no significant differences
Swanson et al., 2006	NS	mph = NS	growth suppression, weight loss
Waring & Lapane, 2008	5-17	Mph	weight loss
Biederman, Spencer, Monuteaux & Faraone, 2010	6-17	mph, dex =NS	no significant difference
Faraone & Mick, 2010	6-13	Dex	weight loss, height gain
Moungnoi & Maipang, 2011	8,6	Mph 0,41-0,49 mg/kg	no significant difference

Glossary: mph=methylphenidate; dex=dextroamphetamine; amx=atomoxetine; NS=not specified.

Spencer, Biederman and Wilens in 1998 reported that the key factor in growth changes depends on the type of treatment. [247] Additionally, he was one the first researchers who stated the hypothesis that growth deficit may not be a direct result of treatment but is in fact a manifestation of ADHD. This hypothesis was also supported by other authors. [213, 211]

Despite the volume of research on growth changes and medication in ADHD, the evidence to support the relationship remains unclear and several studies contain limitations in their methodology. For example, Poulton in 2005 compared 29 studies about children, adolescents, and adults where he found inconsistencies in methodology and findings of the studies. [206] Poulton specifically identified the limited duration of studies, broad age distribution, and a lack of selected parameters (e.g., in determining a physical component it was observed that BMI values did not correspond to appropriate parameters for children, a complete lack of biological age assessment, heritable growth potential in a child was not taken into account, etc.).

Due to the inconsistency of results and a lack of available studies, especially longitudinal studies that analyze growth changes in children who are not medicated, we cannot effectively state whether medication has an effect on growth. The result of monitoring the effect of treatment was compared to the normal population which may have distorted the fact that the disorder itself can be accompanied by physical changes. Today's research shows that the pharmacological treatment of ADHD may not be the main factor that affects growth changes. [211] Finally, a very important observation is that changes in height and weight may happen in children with ADHD regardless of treatment.

4.3.3. Effects of Treatment on the Growth Hormone

The characteristics and nature of growth delay in patients with ADHD is not well understood today. In most cases, the changes in growth are generally not significant enough to warrant a pediatrician to further investigate any additional endocrine assessment. [103] However, cases exist where significant growth changes occur which require an investigation into growth hormone therapy. Children with ADHD who received only growth hormone treatment did not respond well. This suggests that ADHD treatment might in fact contradict growth hormone therapy. [225]

Rao, Julius, Breen and Blethen in 1998 hypothesized that dopamine influences growth hormone secretion. [219] The results of experiments in

ADHD patients with idiopathic growth hormone deficiency (IGDH) who were treated with stimulants such as methylphenidate and pemoline showed the drugs had a significant effect on growth.

Table 5. Effects of growth hormone on growth in patients with ADHD. [103]

Reference	Patient Population	Treatment Status	Study Parameters	Results (SD)
Rao, Julius, Breen & Blethen, 1998	Patients with idiopathic growth hormone deficiency treatment simultaneously for ADHD vs. patients without ADHD	Methylphenidate or pemoline in ADHD	Pre-growth hormone treatment height	– 2.8 ± 0.7 (ADHD) vs. – 3.0 ± 0.9 (non- ADHD)
		Methylphenidate or pemolinein ADHD plus growth hormone	Change in height after growth hormone treatment	1.2 ± 0.8 (ADHD) vs. 1.3 ± 0.9 (non-ADHD)
	Patients with idiopathic small/little growth treated simultaneously for ADHD vs. patients without ADHD	Methylphenidate or pemolinein ADHD	Pre-growth hormone treatment height	– 2.8 ± 0.7 (ADHD) vs. – 2.9 ± 0.7 (non-ADHD)
		Methylphenidate or pemoline in ADHD plus growth hormone	Change in height after growth hormone treatment	1.0 ± 0.7 (ADHD) vs. 1.1 ± 0.7 (non-ADHD)
Frindik, Fowlkes, Kemp, Thrailkill, Morales & Dana, 2009	Patients with idiopathic growth hormone deficiency treatment simultaneously for ADHD vs. patients without ADHD	Stimulant treatment in ADHD	Pre-growth hormone treatment growth rate (cm/year)	3.8 ± 1.8 (ADHD) vs. 4.4 ± 2.3 (non-ADHD)
		Stimulant treatment in ADHD plus growth hormone	Growth rate after one year of growth hormone treatment(cm/year)	8.5 ± 2.0 (ADHD) vs. 9.4 ± 2.6 (non-ADHD)
	Patients with idiopathic small/little growth treated simultaneously for ADHD vs. patients without ADHD	Stimulant treatment in ADHD	Pre-growth hormone treatment growth rate (cm/year)	4.1 ± 1.9 (ADHD) vs. 4.4 ± 2.0 (non-ADHD)
		Stimulant treatment in ADHD plus growth hormone	Growth rate after one year of growth hormone treatment (cm/year)	8.1 ± 1.9 (ADHD) vs. 8.6 ± 2.1 (non-ADHD)
Rose, Reeves, Gut & Germak, 2011	Patients receiving up to 3 years of growth hormone treatment and patients receiving additional ADHD treatment	Stimulant treatment in ADHD vs. non-ADHD patients receiving growth hormone treatment	Change in height after 3 years of growth hormone treatment	1.14 ± 0.60 (ADHD +GH) vs. 1.26 ± 0.79 (non-ADHD)

Frindik, Fowlkes, Kemp, Thrailkill, Morales and Dana in 2009 reported medication treatment of ADHD does not exclude growth hormone treatment. [103] He monitored children receiving treatment for ADHD who had been prescribed growth hormone therapy. (Frindik utilized the national registry of patients treated with the growth hormone). He investigated any differences in anthropometrics and biochemical testing between children with ADHD and children without ADHD. He further compared growth response in children receiving growth hormone therapy only to those receiving growth hormone therapy plus treatment for ADHD. He did not find any differences in the hypothalamic-pituitary-growth hormone axis activity in non-ADHD as compared to those with ADHD. The BMI values did not show any significant changes either. The growth velocity in non-ADHD children was higher at the beginning of the growth hormone treatment as well as after a year of the treatment.

Rose, Reeves, Gut and Germak in 2011 studied patients who received growth hormone therapy for 3 years and found lower height in patients who were also treated with stimulants. [225] After 3 years of growth hormone treatment ADHD patients without the use of stimulants achieved a height greater than patients who received stimulants.

Table 5 summarizes the above mentioned studies.

Based on the above studies, stimulant use appears to influence the growth hormone treatment. Further research is needed to uncover how the process functions and to prove the use of stimulants has a direct influence on the growth hormone. Unfortunately, at this time there are not enough studies to adequately interpret current findings.

4.4. Summary

Physical development and changes in height and weight in children with ADHD are among the most discussed topics among clinicians studying ADHD. Despite the attention received, the causes and associations between ADHD and growth are still not clear.

Children with ADHD can achieve lower physical growth rates while having higher BMI values and a greater proportion of fat in their adipose tissue. The stimulant use is associated with increased occurrences with lower growth rates in both height and weight. However, researchers today believe growth changes occurring during pharmacological treatment are not as significant as was previously believed.

Chapter 5

Variability of Mental Development in ADHD

Abstract

This chapter discusses the variability of mental development in ADHD and emphasizes the characteristics of the developmental and social aspects of ADHD. Attention is one of the main diagnostic criteria of ADHD. However except from diagnostics symptoms, ADHD is associated with a number of other characteristics. Individuals with ADHD face various difficulties in cognitive, emotional, social, sensomotor, and behavioral areas as well as in the process of adaptation. Other characteristic features associated with it are poor memory and executive functions deficit. Children with ADHD lack the ability to strategize and organize information so it can be stored properly and therefore suffer from a weakened working memory.

5.1. Cognitive Development

ADHD is characterized by impaired cognitive development. [165]
The cognitive system is divided into several areas:

- Memory
- Attention and concentration
- Speed of information processing

- Executive function - planning, organizing, problem solving, emotional self-regulation
- Verbal skills and understanding speech
- Spatial orientation and perception

Specific cognitive characteristics are associated with ADHD, such as **attention** (which is one of the key diagnostic criteria of the disorder), **executive dysfunction**, **poor memory, and impaired achievement.**

5.1.1. Attention and concentration

Scientific literature describes differences with individual aspects of **attention**. For example, Vagnerova in 2001 distinguishes aspects of attention in the following way: 1. concentration, 2. tenacity (duration of concentration), 3. distribution (capacity of attention), 4. vigilance, and 5. selectivity. [267]

In individuals with ADHD different aspects of attention are impaired with the primary impairment being the ability to maintain attention. [82] Vagnerova in 2001 on the other hand describes attention impairment in all the areas (tenacity, capacity, vigilance, and selectivity) whereas Paclt, Ptacek and Florian in 2006 and Paclt in 2007 reported problems with endurance and effort. [267, 199, 195]

Barkley in 1997 describes impaired regulatory mechanisms as the primary cause of impaired response inhibition with poor sustained attention being secondary. [22] Impaired ability or inability to concentrate is according to Barkley a secondary cause of impaired response inhibition. Impaired ability to concentrate is also associated with impulsivity. He later identifies differences between individual ADHD subtypes. [23] Those who have difficulties primarily with attention belong in the combined type and those with difficulties with selective attention belong in the inattentive type.

Impaired achievement is another characteristic of ADHD. This impairment can be inconsistent and can manifest itself in many ways e.g., grades or knowledge (a student learns something one day but can not remember it the next day). Research documented these impairments by using standardized tests that measured reaction time. Despite the child's continued efforts he is unable to achieve any consistent results. [62]

5.1.2. Memory

Difficulties with attention can indicate **memory** problems. The individual must first pay close attention to the information before it can be stored in their memory. Recalling the information would require the individual to store it in an organized manner which can be extremely problematic for individuals with ADHD because they lack the strategy and ability to organize. Even if the individual possesses certain information they will not be able to recall it without some level of external assistance or memory jogging by another person.

Children with ADHD achieve variable and inconsistent results during tasks that involve short-term memory. ADHD is further associated with deficits in working memory (e.g., the ability to store information and process it at the same time). Poor **working memory** is one of the characteristics of ADHD. There is a significant variability in how quickly children with ADHD are able to complete tasks using working memory compared to their peers whom do not have ADHD. [97, 50]

Children with ADHD can often remember the same information as non ADHD children but the problem is in their ability to select and identify the important information. They also struggle with planning and decision making. [53]

5.1.3. Executive dysfunction

The name along the understanding of the disorder has changed and today research mainly focuses on hyperactive behavior. The disorder was first viewed as being caused by inappropriate behavior, than there was an alteration in the hypothesis which made it a cognitive disorder leading to maladaptive behavior in terms of attention deficit, impulsivity, and hyperactivity.

Executive function involves a set of mental processes responsible for operating and controlling cognitive, emotional, and behavioral functions especially in activities such as solving new problems. **Executive function** is a term used to describe inter-related functions responsible for planning, setting goals, and problem solving. Specific sub-domains of executive functions consist of a set of controlling or managing functions that include an ability to initiate a specific behavior, suppress other behavior or stimuli, select appropriate goals, plans, organize, and solve complex problems, change problem-solving strategy, and when it is needed assess one's behavior.

Barkley et al. in 1997 described a model of executive dysfunctions located in the prefrontal cortex that explain the cognitive deficits and behavior changes associated with ADHD. [22] His model is constructed from five key executive functions: ability to inhibit, nonverbal working memory, self regulation of emotions and motivation, and reconstitution. The ability to inhibit and exert self-control allows an individual to control verbal and motoric impulses. Non-verbal working memory together with verbal working memory helps the individual to understand what was read. They also play a role in the development of the self-regulation of emotions and motivation as well as moral behavior. Reconstitution helps individuals analyze experience and draw new conclusions from them.

Inhibition control (e.g. the ability to refrain from specific behavior, or not to act impulsively) and ability to stop owns own behavior when the time is appropriate is, according to Barkley in 1990, the fundamental deficit in patients with ADHD and especially in the hyperkinetic-impulsive type (as described in the Diagnostic and Statistical Manual of Mental Disorders, 4th revision (DSM-IV, 1994). [21, 10] Inhibition control also causes other executive dysfunctions, such as a significant inability to adequately direct the necessary attention to achieving goals (behavior analysis, planning, self-regulation, motivation and plan realization). [23]

Individuals with ADHD often exhibit executive deficits during testing and in daily life. These deficits include poor planning, ability to create a strategy, limited organizational abilities, limited self-control (e.g., talking to one-self, often aloud), and poor modulating of emotions (e.g., emotional liability).

In individuals with ADHD, impaired executive functions usually cover more functioning areas than those previously described. Most children, adolescents, and adults with ADHD experience problems in these six areas of impairment to a degree greater than persons without ADHD. [44]

5.1.4. Verbal Skills and Understanding Speech

Patients who have difficulty with verbal skills and understanding speech are often suffering from some form of a psychiatric disorder. [61]

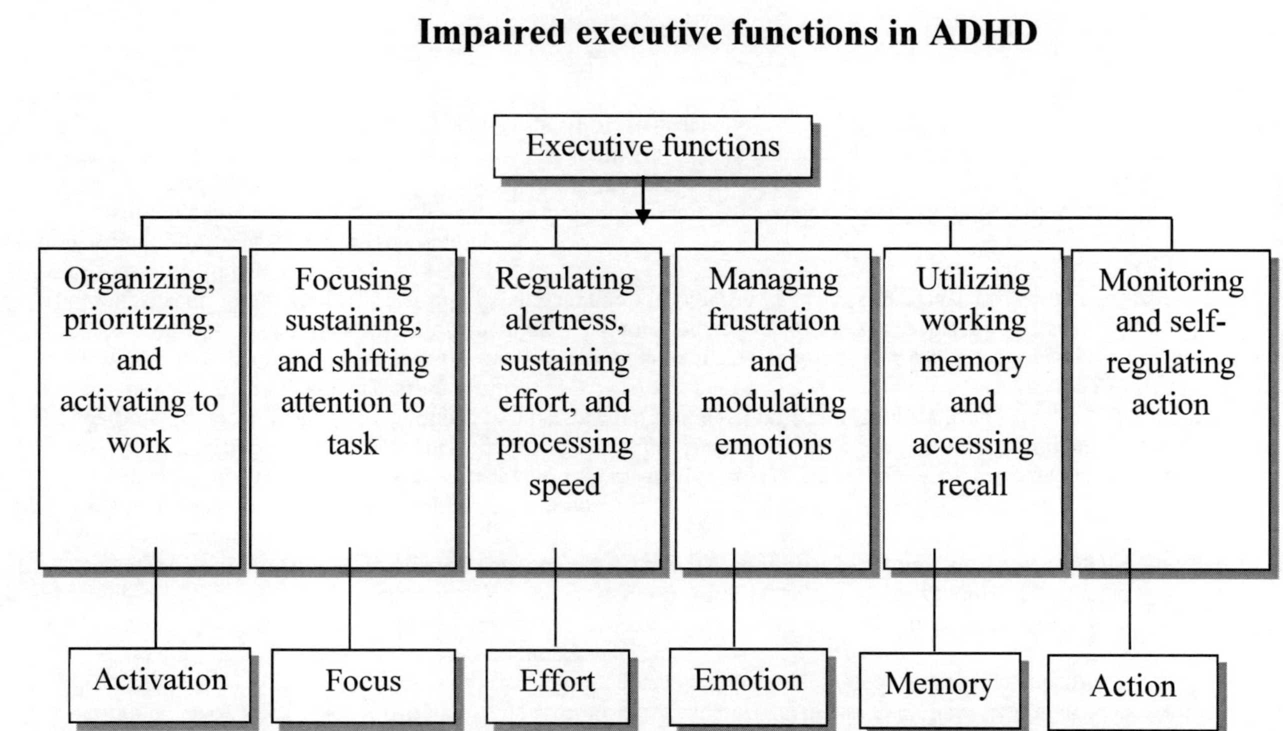

Figure 3. Model of impaired executive functions in ADHD [44].

Activation – organizing tasks and materials, estimating time, prioritizing tasks, and getting started on work tasks.

Individuals with ADHD have difficulty with procrastination, and delay a task they recognize as very important until the very last minute.

Focus – focusing, sustaining focus, and shifting focus to another task.

Some individuals say they are distracted easily not only by things that are going on around them, but also by thoughts in their own mind. Many have reading difficulties as a result of an inability to focus. They generally understand words as they read, but often have to read over and over again in order to fully grasp the meaning of words and to remember them.

Effort – regulating activity, sustaining effort, and processing speed.

Many individuals with ADHD can perform short-term projects well, but have more difficulty with sustained effort over longer periods of time. They find it difficult to complete tasks on time, especially when required to do expository writing. Many also experience chronic difficulty regulating sleep and alertness. These individuals often sleep for a long periods of time or remain awake for extended periods.

Emotion – managing frustration and modulating emotions.

Although the DSM-IV does not recognize criteria related to the management of emotions as an aspect of ADHD, many individuals with this disorder describe difficulties managing frustration, anger, worry, disappointment, desire, and other emotions. They find it difficult to get their emotions into perspective and to get on with what they need to do.

Memory – utilizing memory and accessing recall.

Very often, people with ADHD may have exceptional memory for things that happened long ago, but great difficulty in being able to remember where they just put something, what they wanted to say or what someone just said to them. They have difficulty holding several things in memory while paying attention to other tasks. They often have problems with remembering information they have previously learned.

Action – monitoring and regulating self-action.

Although many individuals with ADHD report they do not experience direct difficulties with hyperactive behavior, they report problems in regulating their actions. They often are too impulsive in what they say, in the way they think or jump too quickly to conclusions. They also report chronic difficulty in regulating their behavior towards others – they can hurt people by what they say or fail to modify their behavior in response to specific circumstances.

Impaired reading and writing is often comorbid with ADHD and it can be difficult to differentiate between comorbid diagnoses and symptoms of ADHD. Children with ADHD have problems with verbal skills, understanding (mostly semantic language - meaning of words), and reading. This is likely because ADHD impairs verbal working memory, attention, and impulsivity. [111] Gremillion and Martel in 2012 state impairment in language and working memory are directly associated with reading problems which leads to academic underachievement. [111]

5.1.5. Spatial Coordination and Perception

Individuals with ADHD may have difficulty with their **motor coordination** and can be described as "clumsy". Their movements are often disorganized and almost one third of them exhibit poor coordination. [99] Children with ADHD can also experience problems with spatial and body orientation. Buderath et al. in 2009 reported subjects had significant difficulties walking backwards and impaired memory for rhythm in movement. [45] These children also have more difficulty learning and performing tasks requiring motor function, such as tying shoelaces, throwing a ball or other accurate movement coordination. [133] These behaviors can manifest until puberty. [99] Related motor deficits were observed also in tasks requiring fine motor skills e.g., dexterity and handwriting. [99]

A significant characteristic of ADHD is excessive motor activity and is generally called hyperactivity. The individual may exhibit erratic and excessive movements, increased mobility not appropriate for circumstances and age (Bedard, Trampush, Newcorn and Halperin), higher rates of involuntary movements, and insufficient hand coordination during task (Klimkeit, Sheppard, Lee and Bradshaw). [28, 140] Some researchers describe varying examples of the incidence of the above mentioned characteristics only in some ADHD subtypes. Mostofsky, Newschaffer and Denckla in 2003 reported occurrences of involuntary movements only in ADHD-combined type. [181] Additionally, Kooistra, Crawford, Dewey, Cantell and Kaplan in 2005 report the impairment of motor functions is more significant in children with the comorbid disorders of Oppositional defiant disorder and dyslexia. [142]

Children with ADHD may also have problems with **visual and auditory perception**. ADHD individuals can experience difficulty "filtering out" irrelevant sensory stimuli from the environment. These children are easily distracted by the sensory stimuli in their environment. This phenomenon is described as "sensory integrative disorder". [17] Additionally, Banaschewski et al. in 2006 found children with ADHD compared to controls experienced distorted color perception. [19] Specific tests showed the distortion occurred along the blue-yellow spectrum (Farnsworth-Munsell 100 Hue Test - FMT) and ADHD children were slower in naming individual colors (Stroop-Color-Word test).

5.2. Social Aspects of ADHD

ADHD is also defined by various shortcomings in the **social settings**. Most individuals with ADHD do not possessa deficit in their social skills and exhibit adequate knowledge about proper social behavior. However, they can fall short in applying their social skills in given situations. When they impulsively enter conversation or play regardless of whether such behavior is socially acceptable, they may appear as inappropriate and annoying. These shortcomings in social behavior can lead to isolation and the individual can be perceived by his peers as awkward and rough. [62]

Individuals with ADHD can have significant difficulty in their social contacts. The problems resulting from their behavior affects their relationships with others and can last throughout their entire life. [268] Vagnerova in 2005 further stated these individuals will probably experience problems in their interpersonal relationships which may increase the likelihood of them failing while trying to socialize. [268]

Individuals with ADHD often achieve lower scores when tested for **adaptation functioning**. The scores are lower not because they do not have sufficient knowledge or lack the ability, but because they fail to apply the skills appropriately. Studies show that when parents provide constant reminders to their children it leads to lower scores in daily functioning testing. [62]

Although the disorder is mostly linked with negative characteristics, there are also several **positive features** that are associated with ADHD. Individuals with ADHD are often more enthusiastic and energetic. They are often very good at creating and developing ideas which are not restricted by traditional boundaries. Although these children often struggle to manage educational programs some adults with ADHD can be very successful in their careers when they can maximize their strength (and minimize their weaknesses). Therefore, it is crucial to support children with ADHD during their school years and help them to focus on their strengths which can be utilized later in life. [62]

There is a significantly small percentage of individuals with ADHD who achieve success in their personal and professional life. These findings are often interpreted in association with ADHD symptoms alone – excessive activity and a frequent shifting of attention. This results in the development of a personality which has dysfunctional characteristics and allows for the individual to absorb and process a significantly higher volume of information than individuals without ADHD. [114] This interpretation gives rise to a fairly interesting premise which cannot be generalized or extended. Further, the prevalence is minute and its interpretation (clinical or statistical) would be burdened by numerous problems interpreting the many variables.

5.3. Developmental Aspects of ADHD

The original view that ADHD starts in childhood and continues till puberty was never scientifically supported. Based on the current research, ADHD is considered a disease that cannot be explicitly cured, starts at an early age, and most likely remains throughout life of the person. Present research shows more and more adolescents carry ADHD symptoms up till adulthood Drtilova and Koukolnik in 1994 reported 30 – 50%. [80] Additionally, Kessler et al. in 2006 reported the prevalence of ADHD in the adult population is almost 4.5%. [135]

When examining adults you can identify characteristics that indicate the presence of ADHD. The characteristics are mostly small deviations, symptoms, or symptom clusters that persisted into adulthood. These dysfunctions worsen over the time due to a myriad of factors – family situation, health status, or because of other stressful situations. [268]

Children with ADHD may fail at work and in social settings when they reach adulthood. [268] Because of their impulsive behavior, men are more likely to get in to a conflict with the law while women are likely to suffer from frequent mood swings or sleep disorders. [24] Some sources even suggest that men who repeatedly committed offenses displayed up to 60 % of the symptoms of ADHD in their medical history. [24] Other symptoms may include an inability to relax, low self-esteem, inability to establish and maintain long-term relationships, increased affectivity, explosivity, etc. [268] ADHD is also associated with a higher frequency of hospitalization, emergency room visits and overall medical costs. [159]

In comparison with children, adults show diminishing hyperactivity which can be attributed to the maturation of CNS. Far more than ever it is necessary to pay attention to impulsivity which in contrast to hyperactivity does not diminish with age but does take on other social contexts.

In many cases difficulties may disappear over time and the child will develop in accordance with the norms. In other times, these difficulties persist throughout childhood until adulthood. However, it cannot be assumed any symptoms will fade away with age. In many cases symptoms will become milder or change, but in about 65 – 80 % of individuals they will persist. [24] Adults with ADHD also achieve a lower socioeconomic status and change their jobs more frequently than adults without ADHD. [24, 268]

Some researchers report the symptoms of ADHD can experience a "fatality" or be abated (Barkley; Paclt and Florian) if a child receives competent and complex treatment (Hallowell and Ratey). [21, 196, 114] With this treatment the symptomatology can significantly be decreased and thus reduce the negative impact the disorder has in adulthood.

5.4. Summary

Despite diagnostic criteria defining ADHD, they do not fully describe the symptoms found in individuals with ADHD. In other words, the diagnosis of ADHD is also associated with a number of other characteristics. Individuals with ADHD face various difficulties in cognitive, emotional, social, sensomotor, and behavioral areas as well as in the process of adaptation.

Attention is one of the main diagnostic criteria of ADHD. Other characteristic features associated with it are poor memory and executive functions deficit. Children with ADHD lack the ability to strategize and organize information so it can be stored properly and therefore suffer from a weakened working memory. For these reasons, their school performance is inconsistent, they continually fail at school and later at work, and their social interactions are negatively impacted.

Chapter 6

Variability of Eating Habits in Children with ADHD

Abstract

This chapter discusses possibly specific eating habits in ADHD patients and mentioned comorbid eating disorders in ADHD petients. According to studies almost half of obese adults meet the diagnostic criteria for ADHD. Symptoms of ADHD are significantly associated with overeating and uncontrolled overeating can cause children with ADHD to become obese or overweight. Individuals with eating disorders share similar characteristics as individuals with ADHD. The common characteristic of both disorders is impulsivity. Impulsivity and decreased self-control may be the causes of patients with ADHD being overweight and obese. Weak inhibitory control and a deficit in executive functioning may also lead to food consumption without the hunger feeling and ultimately end in uncontrollable overeating.

6.1. Introduction

Patients with ADHD are often overweight or obese when compared to non-ADHD individuals. [26] As already mentioned, the incidence of a higher percentage of obese individuals who were unsuccessful at losing weight may be explained by their decreased self-control in their eating habits (Altafas; Curtin, Bandini, Perrin, Tybor and Must) as well as to their abnormal eating patterns and their overall lifestyle (Cortese, Bernardina and Mouren; Cortese et al.). [2, 71, 67, 66] Poor inhibition control and deficits in executive functions which are characteristics of ADHD can also lead to excessive consumption of food. [259, 38, 200] Obesity and ADHD can share similar features as impulsivity and can reflect current basic neurobiological dysfunctions. [66]

According to Altafas in 2002 almost half of obese adults meet the diagnostic criteria for ADHD. [2] Strimas, Davis, Patte, Curtis, Reid and McCool in 2008 found that symptoms of ADHD were significantly associated with overeating. [259] Similarly, Pagoto et al. in 2009 reports that uncontrolled overeating can cause children with ADHD to become obese or overweight. [200] According to Waxman in 2009 the common characteristic of both disorders is impulsivity. [276] Highly impulsive individuals have more difficulty controlling food cravings which leads to higher food intake and predisposes them to obesity. [113] Impulsive children maintain a diet which is far richer in calories compared to the children who do not exhibit impulsive behavior. These children have difficulty delaying their needs and choose food that is easily accessible and readily available e.g., fast food which are high in sugar and fat. [112, 78] Food with appealing taste to the individual can lead to overeating and model addictive behavior. [75] The causes of some cases of obesity may also be attributed to a food addiction. [273] Another hypothesis offered by Davis et al. in 2008 states food can "cure" the hypo dopaminergic condition in ADHD. [76]

According to recent studies and clinical practices the use of stimulants can decrease the appetite and increase weight loss. [208] Medicated children with ADHD were found to have a low percentage of body fat (Ptacek, Kuzelova, Paclt and Zukov; Ptacek, Kuzelova and Paclt), a greater ability to lose weight (Spencer, Faraone, Biederman, Lerner, Cooper and Zimmerman), and a height measurement that was generally lower than the average (Poulton and Nanan). [212, 211, 249, 208] Contraindication exists in stimulant treatments involving patients with low body weight, especially females with anorexia. However, decreased appetite and increased weight loss during treatment can also be caused by alleviating some of the symptoms of ADHD which can further lead to the alleviation of impulsivity while eating. However, these associations still need to be proved. In the end, the question of why individuals with ADHD are in a higher risk category for being overweight and obese is yet to be truly understood.

6.2. ADHD and Comorbid Eating Disorders

Eating disorders include the disorders of anorexia nervosa and bulimia nervosa which are also serious psychiatric disorders and are often comorbid with ADHD. [201]

Patients who suffer from ADHD and eating disorders share similar characteristics such as impulsivity, low self-worth, and neuropsychological features; which includes attention deficit and executive functions. [189, 233] Weak inhibitory control and a deficit in executive functioning may lead to food consumption without the hunger feeling and ultimately end in uncontrollable overeating. [259, 38, 200]

Compounding the understanding the above issues is the literature on ADHD and eating disorders is not very extensive. The reason may be the prevalence of gender differences in both disorders. According to the World Health Organization, the prevalence of overweight and obesity is more frequent in men while eating disorders are more frequent in women (9:1). [174] Additionally, ADHD is more prevalent in boys than in girls. [2]

Davis et al. in 2008 found that symptoms of ADHD are positively correlated with some forms of overeating, such as consumption of food because of bad mood compensation or impact of other negative circumstances. [76]

In this context, women with ADHD are more at risk in the development of eating disorders, especially with bulimia nervosa. [189] Some studies report women with ADHD have a 3.6 times higher chance of developing eating disorders and that ADHD occurs in almost 17% female patients with eating disorders. [32] The ADHD comorbidity was also found in anorexia nervosa (3%) and bulimia nervosa (9%). [38] Additionally, Surman, Randall and Biederman in 2006 reported bulimia nervosa in ADHD patients is more prevalent in adult women than in children or adolescents. [261]

Genetic studies also describe the association between ADHD and eating disorders. Davis and Carter in 2009 pointed at the role the D3 receptor gene plays in ADHD and binge eating. [75] The role of the gene variant in serotonin transporter was repeatedly described in ADHD as well as in eating disorders. [167, 210]

Today, the causal relationship between eating disorders and ADHD has not been fully explained and is still unclear. These relations, however, can have a great clinical and therapeutic significance. Furthermore, it could help clarify changes in physical parameters in children with ADHD – higher prevalence of overweight and obesity and the greater percentage of body fat.

Impulsivity in food consumption in individuals with ADHD can lead to higher caloric intake and can mimic addictive behavior. Individuals with ADHD can exhibit poor planning skills including meal planning and will eat what is currently and quickly available.

There are several possibilities why eating disorders (pathological and non-pathological) occur at a higher rate in patients with ADHD. One reason may be that ADHD and eating disorders share a similar neurobiological foundation.

6.3. Summary

Literature makes an effort to describe the differences in eating habits between individuals with ADHD and individuals without ADHD in relation to the higher prevalence of overweight and obesity in patients with ADHD. It is reported that impulsivity and decreased self-control may be the causes of patients with ADHD being overweight and obese. Individuals with eating disorders share similar characteristics as individuals with ADHD. Weak inhibitory control and a deficit in executive functioning may also lead to food consumption without the hunger feeling and ultimately end in uncontrollable overeating. Literature states that almost 9 % of patients with ADHD also suffer from bulimia nervosa. The causal relationship between eating disorders and ADHD remains unclear. These relations, however, can likely have a great clinical and therapeutic significance.

Chapter 7

Variability in Treatment of ADHD

Abstract

This chapter provides information about the treatment available for ADHD. It introduces pharmacotherapy, mechanism of treatment and the possible presence of side effects. There are metioned psychopharmacological approach (stimulants and non-stimulants) and behavioral /psychosocial approach in this chapter. There is compared efficacy of methods, effects as well as side effects. This chapter emphasizes the fact that treatment of ADHD essentially improves the individuals functioning in his social and professional area. This section has been also inserted to discuss the topic of pharmacotherapy in ADHD in terms of choosing the appropriate drug, understanding the side effects of the drugs, and to analyze the physical development and body growth that occurs through the process.

7.1. Treatment Methods

Although ADHD is not a disorder that would threaten the child's life it does, however, take away his ability to successfully engage in social interactions. It is reported that up to 80% of untreated individuals carry symptoms through adulthood. Individuals who do not receive any treatment are unable to apply their skills in life situations and their interactions with peers are problematic. Such an individual is often lonely because his peers reject him and the individual experiences a personal frustration due to his setbacks in these settings. [164-165] In adulthood individuals with ADHD are at a higher risk of being diagnosed with other disorders e.g., Conduct disorders, Antisocial personality disorder, Substance use disorder, and additional problems in social relationships. [77]

Treatment of ADHD is therefore crucial. With proper treatment the child has a greater chance to develop his skills and achieve the adequate social and professional status in the future. [77]

Like the treatment of all pediatric psychiatric disorders, ADHD treatment also includes cooperation with the doctor (especially the child psychiatrist, and psychologist), parents, and teachers. There are several methods and procedures used in ADHD treatment with each having a greater or lesser efficacy. The ADHD treatment focuses on the following approaches of treatment:

1. Pharmacological approach
2. Behavioral/Psychosocial approach
3. Combination of approaches

Hrdlicka in 2007 states that a very high percentage of children are treated inappropriately or are not treated at all. [123] The reasons for this may be the problem in assessing the correct diagnoses and choosing the proper treatment method. Furthermore, these problems likely occur due to diagnostic errors, especially when the disorder is influenced by comorbid disorders (incorrect use of diagnosis, frequent changes in the concept of diagnosis), unsuitable choice of treatment (overuse of neuroleptics), and preference of psychotherapy before pharmacotherapy, etc.

Based on the current views the most efficient treatment methods for ADHD are pharmacotherapy, psychotherapeutic techniques, and the combination of the two. [81, 83] It cannot be said which of these methods is more effective and the treatment always depends on each individual and the selected approach the clinician takes in addressing the patient's needs. Longitudinal studies on the effectiveness of different types of treatment (behavioral therapy, combination of medication and behavioral therapy, and medication only) showed that after 8 years of research all individuals who received some kind of treatment improved with no significant difference improvement between the groups. [179]

However, it was found in the meta-analysis of 74 studies performed by Purdie, Hattie and Carroll that the pharmacological approach was the most significant treatment avenue for behavior but the least effective in the educational processes. [215] The study ultimately illustrates the significance educational approaches have upon academic performance over the use of medication or psychotherapy.

The American Academy of Pediatrics states the methods to be used as the first choice to treat ADHD are behavioral therapy, medication, and self-verbalization. They do not find Cognitive Behavioral Therapy (CBT) or parental training to be effective.

The following table presents levels of support in individual treatment methods for ADHD according to the American Academy of Pediatrics - mental health.

Table 6. Levels of support in treatment methods for ADHD [5]

Level 1 **Best support**	**Level 2** **Good support**	**Level 3** **Moderate support**	**Level 4** **Minimal support**	**Level 5** **No support**
• Behavioral therapy • Medication • Self-verbalization	• Biofeedback • Contingency Management • Education • Parental training in coping skills /management (alone with Problem solving, or with Psychoeducation of teachers) • Exercise • Relaxation and exercise • Social skills and medication • Work memory training	---	• Parental training in coping skills and social skills • Relaxation • Self-verbalization and Contingency Management • Social skills	• Attention • Client - centered therapy • CBT • CBT and anger management • Parental training in coping skills/stress management • Parental training in coping skills and Self-verbalization • Problem solving • Training in self-control • Self-verbalization and medication • Skills development

Note: Level 5 refers to forms of treatment that tests assessed as not supportive or their efficacy was not proved/ was inconclusive.

It is important to stress that none of the treatment methods permanently eliminate the symptoms of ADHD, it only suppresses them. The treatment brings temporary relieve only for the time that it is applied. Once the treatment ends, the same symptoms that were present before the start of the treatment frequently return. This suppression factor is an outstanding characteristic feature of pharmacotherapeutical procedures. [24]

7.2. Psychotherapy

Psychotherapy offers a wide range of treatment options and includes behavioral therapy, special social training and traditional or group therapy. Psychotherapy consists of interviews conducted by a psychotherapist with the child and his family. The goal of psychotherapy is to strengthen the mutual cooperation, teach the child to cope with the ADHD symptoms, increase the self-esteem of the child, and improve his communication with others. The psychotherapist provides consultations to parents and teachers which are focused on imprinting certain behavior patterns that would support adaptation abilities, positive reactions, and improvement in academic performance. This method supports systematic changes in routines as it relates to family and the school environment so the child functions better. This means organizing time and places, division of tasks, and motivating the child.

Cognitive Behavioral Therapy is appropriate especially when:

- Stimulant medication is only partially effective or not effective at all, and as a combination with medication.
- The patient has difficulty accepting the ADHD diagnosis and the associated pharmacotherapy.
- The patient has a comorbid diagnoses, for example; Anxiety disorder or depression.
- Psychological care is sufficient to alleviate the symptoms and functional impairment.

Therapy focuses on training in behavioral skills, especially developing a strategy to cope with the ADHD symptoms and desirable behavior training.

Behavioral therapy in ADHD treatment is a significant method in many respects. Children with ADHD are inattentive, hyperactive, and impulsive which causes difficulties in everyday activities at school, peer acceptance, social relationships, and family environment. The way the child addresses these problems determines his future success or failure. The way in which the child will function in adulthood is predetermined by how efficiently his parents apply their parenting skills in coaching the child, how he gets along with peers, and how well he does at school. Psychotherapy is not solely focused on the child but also helps educate teachers and parents how to help the child cope with the disorder. Mastering these skills is essential because they can be utilized throughout the individual's whole life. [277]

Efficacy

Although psychotherapy does not receive the same empirical support as pharmacotherapy does, its efficacy is indisputable. While medication can suppress neurobiological symptoms of the disorder, in a number of individuals it is not efficient or some residual symptoms may occur. Medication does not focus on every area of an individual's functioning. [141]

The most efficient treatment is a comprehensive approach with psychotherapy and pharmacotherapy overlapping where they can be complemented by certain lifestyle changes and educational measures.

7.3. Psychopharmacology

As already mentioned, pharmacotherapy is one of the most successful methods used to treat ADHD. A series of studies demonstrated that the use of stimulants (methylphenidate and dextroamphetamine) and non-stimulants (atomoxetine) have a positive effect on the symptoms of ADHD. [31]

Prior to the initiation of the treatment and regardless of the choice of the medication the patient uses, clinician needs to completely asses the child. This assessment involves an internal and neurological examination, laboratory tests, psychological tests, information from the school and a detailed interview with the parents and child. At the beginning of the treatment the clinician needs to identify the goals of the treatment. Pharmacological treatment must then be chosen based on the in-depth evaluation and the medication must always be part of a complete care package which consists of psychosocial, behavioral, and educational intervention.

7.3.1. Stimulants

The most common medications used to treat ADHD are the stimulants methylphenidate, dextroamphetamine, and pemoline. At this moment only methylphenidate is used to treat ADHD in the Czech Republic. Methylphenidate is also the most common stimulant used in the world to treat ADHD. The most frequently prescribed drugs from the methylphenidate group are its short-acting form Ritalin (biological half-lifee 2.5 hours, clinical effects last for about 2.5-4 hours) and its long-acting form Concerta (clinical effects 10-12 hours).

Mechanism of Action

Stimulants block the activities of dopamine transporter, reuptake dopamine, and noradrenaline in the presynaptic neurons. They also increase the release of neurotransmitters from the synaptic cleft. Additionally, stimulants cause a response delay and affect the working memory. [272]

Efficacy

Almost 70% of patients with ADHD have positive effects from the use of stimulants (American Academy of Child and Adolescent Psychiatry; Maidment) even during long-term treatment (Charach, Ickowicz and Schachar). [4, 163, 56] The effects of stimulants are almost immediate, but the effective duration is short-lived and frequent use is needed to alleviate the symptoms of ADHD.

Effects

Stimulants activate the effect of catecholamine and lead to the increase of dopamine levels which acts on motor coordination and also increase noradrenaline levels. Stimulants cause the excitation of the respiratory center in the medulla and stimulate the reticular activating system which causes improved attention, motivation, and decreased tiredness. Therefore, this process ultimately leads to improved school performance (school tasks). They can significantly contribute to the improvement in the conditions of attention deficit, impulsivity, hyperactivity, aggressiveness, and disobedience. They also stimulate attention, memory, learning, increase accuracy at work, and decrease the number of errors. They also alleviate socially inappropriate behaviors connected with excessive movements which then lead to less peer rejections.

Stimulants effects can be divided the following way:

- *Effects on cognition* – improves attention, short-term memory, reduces restlessness and impulsivity, improves ability to finish work once it begins, improves accuracy.
- *Effects on motor skills* – decreases hyperactivity, improves fine motor skills (motion accuracy, dexterity).
- *Effects on social skills* – improves social acceptance among peers, inhibits anger affects, verbal and physical aggression, diminishes impulsive urge to destroy things, reduces defiance and oppositional behavior, improves the ability to play independently.

Side Effects

The most common reported side effects of methylphenidate are loss of appetite, stomach pain, nausea, headaches, nervous feeling, sleep problems, growth delay, and growth suppression. [56, 94] Some of the side effects are only temporary however, it is quiet common that they can remain throughout the treatment. [56]

Animal models show methylphenidate likely delays the development of the testicles when administered in the pre-pubertal stage. [169] Despite the initial delay, observations after 40 months revealed testicular volume and testosterone production returned to normal levels.

Similarly, amphetamine also reduces certain phases of sleep. It affects the satiety center in the hypothalamus and decreases the appetite in children treated for ADHD. The stimulants do have side effects and predominantly target the cardiovascular system. Methylphenidate evokes a small but significant change in blood pressure and heart rate with higher doses causing a possible arrhythmia.

Research shows that long-term use of medication in childhood increases the risk for substance abuse up to 50%. [230] The question whether stimulant use has any significant long-term effects (positive or negative) has still not been proven. [77]

Current literature states that long-term use of stimulants may cause reduced efficiency. Fusar-Poli, Rubia, Rossi, Sartori and Balottin in 2012 found that people who never used stimulants previously exhibited a significantly lower dopamine transporter levels than people who sometimes used stimulants. [104] A higher density of dopamine transporters in the striatum in these individuals is probably a compensatory mechanism resulting from the higher dopamine levels in the brain.

7.3.2. Non-stimulants

Atomoxetine

Since 2003, the non-stimulant medication atomoxetine began to be used to treat ADHD. Both methylphenidate and atomoxetine are the primary medications prescribed with atomoxetine having long-term effects compared to methylphenidate's short-term effects. Since 2007, in the Czech Republic, the primary non-stimulant drug used is Strattera.

Mechanism of Action

Atomoxetine is a central sympathomimetic drug inhibiting reuptake of noradrenaline while also blocks the presynaptic noradrenaline transporter. [148] Atomoxetine increases extracellular levels of dopamine in the prefrontal cortex while modulating cortical synaptic reuptake of dopamine through the noradrenaline transporter. Additionally, treatment with atomoxetine does not have psychostimulant effects. [262]

Efficacy

Short-term and long-term studies show that atomoxetine has a good therapeutic efficacy. This was evidenced in several studies that observed efficacy of certain doses of atomoxetine compared to a placebo. Fewer studies focus on comparisons of atomoxetine and stimulants.

Spencer et al. in 2002 reported that 60% of patients respond positively to treatment with atomoxetine. [250] Michelson et al. in 2002 proved its efficacy [172] While administering the drug to patients once a day and the results did not correspond to elimination half-life, but the clinical experience confirmed longer efficacy.

Some individuals respond well to treatment with methylphenidate as well as to treatment with atomoxetine, however, some of the individuals reported they seem to respond better to one active substance. [60] Banaschewski et al. reported similar efficacy of both types of medication. [19] There is a lack of long-term qualitative studies with large enough samples to prove this and, therefore, definite results cannot be concluded.

Effects

Unlike stimulants, atomoxetine has a full effect after four weeks of usage and does not have the one dosage effect. [123] It differs from stimulants with its continual influence on symptoms of ADHD, including sleep disorders, and can be administered once a day. It effects cognitive and psychosocial functions, improves attention, and decreases impulsivity, hyperactivity, restlessness, and aggression. It leads to better results at school, improves acceptance from parents and peers, and improves social relationships. The above mentioned effects increaseself-worth and self-esteem of the patient. [27]

Effects of atomoxetine can be divided the following way:

- *Effects on cognition* – improves attention and short-term memory, alleviation of restlessness and impulsivity, improves task completion and accuracy.

- *Effects on motor skills*– decreases hyperactivity, improves fine motor skills (motion accuracy, dexterity).
- *Effects on social skills* – improves social status among peers, inhibits anger affects, verbal and physical aggression, reduce impulsive urge to destroy things, defiance and oppositional behavior, improves ability to play independently.

Table 7. Comparison of common side effects of ADHD medication

Drug	Mechanism of action on molecular level	Common side effects	References
Methylphenidate	Blocks reuptake of dopamine and reuptake of noradrenaline, blocks dopamine transporter	Decreased appetite, insomnia, stomach pain, headache and dizziness, weight loss, affective symptoms, nausea, vomiting, insomnia, anorexia	Faraone, Pucci & Coghill, 2009a; Faraone, 2009b; Biederman, Mick, Wozniak, Monuteaux, Galdo & Faraone, 2003b
Dextroamphetamine	Increases release of dopamine and noradrenaline into synaptic cleft, decreases reuptake	Decreased appetite, insomnia, palpitation, tremor, headache, dizziness, dry mouth, weight loss, abdominal symptom, stomach pain, irritability	Faraone, Pucci & Coghill, 2009a; Faraone, 2009b; Curatolo, D´Agati & Moavero, 2010
Mixed amphetamine salts	Increases release of dopamine and noradrenaline into synaptic cleft, decreases reuptake	Decreased appetite, agitation, insomnia, headache	Faraone, Pucci & Coghill, 2009a; Faraone, 2009b; Curatolo, D´Agati & Moavero, 2010
Atomoxetine	Selectively inhibits synaptic reuptake of dopamine	Stomach pain, decreased appetite, vomiting, somnolence, irritability, fatigue	Kratochvil, Milton, Vaughan & Greenhill, 2008

Side Effects

The side effects of non-stimulan tuse are generally temporary. The most common side effects are stomach pain, vomiting, and loss of appetite. In other cases individuals can experience early morning awaking, irritation, mood swings, dizziness, drowsiness, constipation, nausea, tiredness, and weight loss.

Treatment with atomoxetine is not associated with a risk for the development of addiction and tics. [83]

Despite the good efficacy of the medication some side effects can occur. Research on methylphenidate and atomoxetine shows there is an influence on blood pressure and heart rate, however, a clear connection has not been established. The following table compares side effects of specific drugs.

7.3.3. Others

Another treatment option for children with ADHD is tricyclic antidepressants. These antidepressants, as well as stimulants, have similar effects on the nervous system. The use of tricyclic antidepressants, however, can cause an increase in blood pressure and acceleration of the heart rate in children but not in adults. Side effects on the cardiovascular system may be significant and certain cardio-toxicity can occur.

Another medication used to treat ADHD and which is used in small dosages are neuroepileptics. The way these neuroepileptics work is also similar to stimulants. The disadvantage of treatment with neuroepileptics is psychomotor retardation and decreased attention. An atypical neuroepileptic drug is Risperidone. Research shows, that Risperidone decreases aggressiveness, irritability, and hyperactivity. It is used especially in cases where the presence of conduct disorders is diagnosed. [85]

7.4. Variability in Response to Treatment

Despite the high efficacy of pharmacotherapy in ADHD there is quiet a high variability in the medication response andfinding the optimal dosage at the onset of the treatment. Consistently stated procedures that predict the response to treatment and which would also determine the optimal dosage are as of yet not established. Decisions about treatment planning are often determined empirically and are based on the clinical experience of the doctor.

The variability in the response to treatment is also highly attributed to genetic factors. These factors are the primary focus of pharmaco-genetic studies but the results of these studies are still undefined and inconsistent.

Table 8. Association between response to treatment and genetic variation

Gene	Variation	Association with response to treatment	Citations
ADRA2A	C1291G SNP	better response in G allele carriers (inattention)	Polanczyk et al., 2007; Da Silva et al., 2008
COMT	Val158Met	better response in homozygous Vallallele carriers	Kereszturi et al., 2008
DAT (SLC6A3)	count 40bp VNTR	decreased response in allele carrier with 9 and 10 repetitions, especially homozygotes 10/10, higher incidence of side effects of treatment in homozygotes 9/9	Cheon, Ryu, Kim & Cho, 2005; Purper-Ouakil et al., 2008; Stein et al., 2005
DRD4	count VNTR	decreased response in allele carriers with 7 repetitions	Joober et al., 2007; McGough et al., 2006; Roman, Szobot, Martins, Biederman, Rohde & Hutz, 2002; Hamarman, Fossella, Ulger, Brimacombe & Dermody, 2004
DRD2, DRD5	one-nucleotide Taq polymorphism	no effect	Winsberg & Comings, 1999
CHRNA4	rs1044396 a rs6090384	no effect	Tharoor, Lobos, Todd & Reiersen, 2008
SLC6A2	G1287A SNP	decreased response for homozygotes A/A	Yang, Wang, Li & Faraone, 2004
HTR1B, HTR2A		no effect	Zeni et al., 2007
5HTT (SLC6A4)	length polymorphism L, S	decreased response in L/L homozygotes in combination with 7/7 for DRD4; no effect	Seeger, Schloss & Schmidt, 2001; Zeni et al., 2007
SNAP25	T1065G a T1069C	decreased incidence of side effects in homozygotes T1065G G (sleep difficulties) and T1069C C homozygotes (tics)	McGough et al., 2006

Variability in response to treatment is not only likely associated with genetic factors but also involves the presence of side effects from the treatment. Some frequently occurring variants associated with ADHD also decrease the response to treatment (e.g., DRD4 allele with 7 repetitions). On the other hand, other variants may enhance treatment success (e.g., ADRA 2A snp A-1291 C > G). Also, in relation to other variants a lower presence of the side effects of treatment, were found to be related to other variants (e.g., SNAP 25 T1065G). Table 8 provides an overview of these associations.

Pharmacogenetic studies help to understand variability in response to treatment in children with ADHD and leads to improving treatment procedures. Existing pharmacogenetic studies, however, are quiet controversial mainly due to different characteristics of individual studies, dosage of the medication, and measurement/observation criteria. Meaningful conclusions and advances in the area of pharmaocogenetics and ADHD would benefit from studies with a sufficiently large sample of propends and the use of standardized testing. Additionally, observing enzymes that metabolize drugs and utilizing a wide spectrum of stimulants and non-stimulants is necessary to make any definite conclusions.

7.5. Summary

ADHD is a disorder that requires a multifactorial treatment. According to current beliefs, the most effective treatment methods for ADHD are pharmacotherapy, psychotherapeutic techniques, and the ideal combination of the two. Psychotherapy helps individuals with ADHD to cope with disorder manifestation, enhances a child's self-esteem, and improves communication with others. Improvement is usually apparent in many areas such as decreased attention, hyperactivity, and aggressiveness, learning effectivity, and better placement within a group. Pharmacological treatment that uses stimulants and non-stimulants significantly increases activation of the key cortical and subcortical brain regions which are associated with attention. [279] Treatment with stimulants and non-stimulants (atomoxetine) improves attention and reduces symptoms of hyperactivity and impulsivity. There is a significant variability in response to treatment which is, for the most part, caused by genetic factors. These associations are still to this day not properly explained.

Treatment of ADHD essentially improves the individuals functioning in his social and professional area. Individuals who are not treated often exhibit symptoms of ADHD until adulthood and these symptoms may result in mental disorders, problems in social life, and failure at work etc.

Chapter 8

ADHD in Adulthood

ABSTRACT

This chapter attends to nowadays very actual topic, which is ADHD in adulthood. The manifestation of ADHD does changes with the transition from childhood to adulthood. The apparent forms are increased emotional lability, irritability, impulsivity, and attention deficits. ADHD symptoms were not viewed as persistent but as a manifestation of another psychopathology. ADHD is not being sufficiently diagnosed in adults today, which is most certainly causing serious problem for adults in social functioning. This chapter provides imńformation about ADHD symptoms, diagnostics and treatment in adulthood and mentioned also comorbidity. It is very important topic because it is estimated that 50 % of cases diagnosed with ADHD in childhood persist through adulthood.

8.1. Introduction

For many years, ADHD was considered a childhood disorder and was only addressed as such in previous DSM manuals. The DSM-5, however, re-defines ADHD as a lifelong disorder that may remain with the individual through childhood into adulthood. Existing studies show that ADHD lasts till adulthood in 50 % of individuals (Goodman & Thase, 2009 [110]) and is prevalent in almost 4 % of the adult population. The manifestation of ADHD does, however, change with the transition from childhood to adulthood. ADHD symptoms were not viewed as persistent but as a manifestation of another psychopathology e.g., Conduct disorders or Affective disorders. In developing the parameters associated with an ADHD prognosis certain unfavorable attributes were considered such as positive family medical history, adverse living conditions, and the incidence of psychiatric comorbidity (Conduct disorders, Defiant oppositional disorder, Anxiety disorders, and Mood disorders). [24]

ADHD is not being sufficiently diagnosed in adults today, which is most certainly causing serious problem for adults in social functioning. Even adults with ADHD can be treated with an effective therapeutic intervention; therefore greater attention should be given to ADHD prevalence and symptoms in adulthood. The relatively new idea that ADHD persists through adulthood and that it can also be diagnosed in adults is accommodated for in the DSM-5.

8.2. Symptoms of ADHD in Adulthood

Symptoms of ADHD are often transmitted from childhood to adulthood in a slightly modified form. The apparent forms are increased emotional liability, irritability, impulsivity, and attention deficits.

Hyperactivity which is a frequent and dominant symptom in childhood recedes in adulthood and takes on a form with different qualitative symptoms such as inner restlessness, increased impulsivity, difficulty to control moods, impatience, and failure to comply with rules (e.g., speed limit when driving), nervousness and the need for instant changes. [24] A symptom that persists in adulthood is attention deficit and it is often discrete and therefore ADHD is often under-diagnosed in adults. Attention deficit in adulthood causes difficulties at work, chaotic lifestyle, forgetfulness, inability to maintain systematic work process, task or problem solving difficulties, and the inability to concentrate on given tasks which leads to their incompletion.

Another dominant symptom of ADHD in adulthood is impulsivity. It affects the ability to plan and make decisions. These adults tend to be impatient and make hasty decisions. They can have difficulty estimating situations and react in adequately. They have problems recognizing socially appropriate reactions, controlling their reactions, respecting conventions and authority.

Adults with ADHD often report difficulties in relationships, higher divorce rates, difficulty working as a team, and frequent conflicts at work. As a result of these difficulties and their constant failures they can feel frustrated and have a low self-worth for lengthy periods. These additional difficulties often lead to the development of Anxiety disorders and depression. [51]

The clinical picture of ADHD in adulthood is extremely complex and it can be difficult to diagnose and effectively treat. Some individuals experience impulsivity, feelings of inner restlessness, and the inability to complete tasks while others have difficulty controlling their mood and problems in social relations. The previously mentioned symptoms were all previously assessed to be indicators of Mood disorders, Neurotic disorders and Personality disorders when in fact these symptoms were related to ADHD as we know it today. The new perspective on ADHD as a lifelong diagnosis can be helpful to suffering adults in many ways. However, it can also lead to it being over diagnosed and therefore the root causes can be overlooked. With the publishing of the manual DSM-5, the long "silence" and the countless questions in respect to ADHD in adulthood are being addressed and the current psychiatric world is changing forever.

8.3. Diagnosis of ADHD in Adulthood

The diagnosis of ADHD in adulthood is based primarily on the clinical evaluation of the current symptomatology and the existing development of the disorder. Both of the previously mentioned clinical practices are indispensable conditions for the ADHD diagnosis. In order to make the appropriate diagnosis it is beneficial to obtain information from people who are close to the patient. [51] The clinical evaluation can be completed by utilizing rating scales designed to test ADHD symptoms in adulthood. These scales include the Conners Adults ADHD Rating Scaleand the Wender Utah Rating Scale (WURS). Furthermore, it s possible to use a series of neuropsychological tests, for example, the Continuous Performance Task (CPT) test or other tests that focus on evaluating attention or related functions such as working memory, executive functions etc. These tests can reveal specific deficits in different areas but they cannot be specifically used to test ADHD in the sense of "cut off scores" etc. In order to effectively diagnose ADHD in adulthood we must further explore this topic in future studies.

8.4. Comorbidity

As already mentioned, ADHD is associated with a higher presence of comorbid diagnoses. Jensen et al. in 2001 report 70 % of individuals with

ADHD suffer from at least one psychiatric disorder. [128] In adulthood, individuals with ADHD suffer usually from Mood disorders, Anxiety disorders, Conduct disorders, and addiction.

According to Murphy and Barkley in 1996, adult ADHD patients have a higher rate of Alcoholism (35 % vs. 10 %), Substance use disorder (14 % vs. 3 %), and Conduct disorders (17 % vs. 0 %). [187] Additionally, 32 % suffer from Anxiety disorders, 18 % suffer from Depressive disorders, and 32 % suffer from dysthymia.

The diagnosis of comorbid disorders can be difficult to make and recognizing comorbid disorders is vital in any psychotherapeutic and pharmacologic interventions. On the other hand, the situation may be reversed where other psychiatric disorders may cause similar changes or manifest similar symptoms as those associated with ADHD. These symptoms can be mistakenly diagnosed as ADHD and therefore they need to be clearly distinguished from ADHD symptoms. For example, Mood disorders and Anxiety disorders include the symptom of decreased attention that exactly mimics the same symptom in ADHD. [86] In many cases it is necessary to make a differential diagnostic decision to decide if the disorder is ADHD or another disorder and chose which disorder is primary and which disorder is secondary. For example, persistent ADHD symptoms can lead to the development of secondary disorders. For example, persistent ADHD symptoms can lead to the development of Mood disorders. Finally, it is important to differentiate if the two disorders (ADHD and its comorbid disorder) occur together.

Treatment of ADHD in Adulthood

Treatment of ADHD in adulthood, as in childhood, focuses on the following three approaches:

1. Pharmacological approach
2. Behavioral/Psychosocial approach
3. Combination of both methods

In the first step the patient is informed about all the aspects of the disorder, individual symptoms, pathophysiology of ADHD and difficulties in various life activities. [108] After informing the patient of the aspects of the conditions an appropriate treatment plan is chosen - pharmacological approach, psychotherapeutic approach or combination of both methods.

8.5.1. Psychotherapy

The most appropriate form of treatment in adult and child patients with ADHD is the Cognitive behavioral therapy which is applied when:

- Psychological care is sufficient to alleviate symptoms and deficits in functioning.
- Medication itself is only partially efficient or not efficient at all.
- Patient has difficulty accepting the diagnosis of ADHD and pharmacotherapy.
- Patient suffers from comorbid diagnoses, for example, Anxiety disorders and depression.

Treatment focuses especially on behavioral skills training like strategy coping with symptoms of ADHD and practice of desirable behaviors. Patients learn to organize daily activities, meet deadlines, and fulfill their obligations.

Using psychotherapy as a method to treat ADHD is very important and efficient in adult patients because medication is not focused on all areas of persons functioning. Medication, however, clearly has more support in the treatment of ADHD. Cognitive behavioral therapy helps patients manage daily responsibilities while training them to employ desirable behavior.

8.5.2. Pharmacotherapy

Based on a series of studies, it was demonstrated that stimulant treatment using methylphenidate and dextroamphetamine, as well as non-stimulant treatment using atomoxetine, has a positive effect on the symptoms of ADHD. [31] The most commonly used pharmacological drugs in childhood and adulthood are stimulants. However, adults with ADHD can experience problems with dosage and the lasting effects of methylphenidate because their difficulty in organizing and planning prevent them from using their medication regularly. An alternative to stimulants is a drug called atomoxetine. Atomoxetine has a longer lasting effect and its efficacy is not influenced by problems with regular use.

8.6. Summary

Although historical research focused mostly on ADHD in childhood it is becoming apparent ADHD represents a serious problem for adults. It is estimated that 50 % of cases diagnosed with ADHD in childhood persist through adulthood and the only changes occurring are symptom manifestations. However, ADHD significantly impairs individual functioning in social and working environment and it is crucial to treat ADHD as a problem than can inflict an individual at any age.

Chapter 9

ADHD As Controversial Diagnosis

Abstract

ADHD is the most diagnosed disorder in childhood and also one of the most researched disorders today. Despite the vast research there are many unanswered questions regarding the diagnosis, differential diagnostics, etiology, treatment and other areas with new question sarising each day. The chapter presents controversial topics about ADHD. The first controverse is diagnosis ADHD itself. Other controvercial topic is etiology of ADHD. Research suggests that genetic factors play an important role in the symptomatology of the disorder but the role of genetics is still unclear. Pharmacology is also very discussed and controversial topic as well as comorbidity. This last chapter opens the question how much is ADHD controversial diagnosis.

9.1. Diagnosis of ADHD

Many researchers agree that a diagnosis of ADHD is controversial. [136, 125] Matejcek, in 2003, points out how problematic it can be to distinguish between pathological conditions and normal conditions to make diagnoses. [168] Creating criteria, some of which may not be present to make a diagnosis, leads to the question of what conditions are pathological and what are normal.

The field of diagnostics has been for decades developing, refining, and narrowing a basis for a diagnosis beginning with the symptoms of non-specific syndromes and working towards the specific manifestations defined in the DSM-5. The diagnosis of ADHD is a summary of the symptoms of the three basic areas of hyperactivity, impulsivity, and inattention. These are non-specific symptoms which are also included in several other psychiatric diagnoses. Therefore, when making a diagnosis of ADHD certain disorders and conditions need to be excluded that would normally also contain these symptoms.

What also seems to be problematic is the over-diagnosing of individuals with ADHD. In many cases, behavior that leads to failure at school is arbitrarily diagnosed as ADHD. However, this behavior can be viewed from two different perspectives. Does the individual really suffer from the disorder or is the "undesirable" behavior associated with the environment that could be changed by making an alteration like placing the child in another class (e.g., a class with fewer students). Society often requires individuals adjust behaviors and adapt to a given order, especially at school or work. For some individuals this comes naturally and they accept and manage such conformity with ease. However, for some people attempting to conform presents numerous difficulties. For some individuals it is practically impossible to handle tasks that are not enjoyable or stimulating. This causes problems with suppression and gives rise to other impulses (talking, movement, attracting the attention of others). Is the ADHD diagnosis a practical answer in these cases? Is ADHD really a psychiatric disorder in the true and literal sense?

In this respect substantiating a diagnosis of ADHD remains problematic. Other disorders posses specific assessment methods that help to diagnose the psychopathological phenomena, but in the case of the ADHD diagnosis this is not possible as of yet. Psychological assessments can contribute to the non-specific diagnosis of attention, executive functions etc. but it does not allow for a specific diagnosis of any ADHD symptoms.

9.2. Etiology of ADHD

The etiology of ADHD is also an area with a great deal of controversy. Similarly to research in other areas of ADHD, studies about the etiological factors of ADHD are limited (e.g., differential methodology, deficient sample, the wide range in the age of the monitored children etc.). For these reasons, there are many questions about etiology that still remain without explanation.

Research suggests that genetic factors play an important role in the symptomatology of the disorder. In this context, the question becomes to what extent is it possible to treat ADHD with drugs? If the drugs have an effect on the symptomatology of ADHD the question remains as to which gene regulations these drugs penetrate. Thapar, Cooper, Eyre and Langley in 2013 reported genetic testing cannot be used to predict ADHD nor can it be used for any diagnostic purposes because the study results on how genetics influence ADHD is controversial despite several studies showing possible linkages. [264] The main reason for the controversy is the number of studies is few and the results are not fully understood. Additionally, genetic participation in ADHD does not necessarily mean that medication is needed to treat the disorder. When ADHD is present in the family (parents and siblings) an intervention involving treatment of some sort for the whole family needs to be considered. At present, too much attention may be paid to genetic factors and their importance in the etiology in ADHD. It is understandable in today's world where the focus on genetics is heightened that research efforts are being directed towards genetics with a subsequent effort to implement genetic testing into the diagnostic process.

Husarova and Ondrejka are concerned with the neurobiological nature in the symptomatology of ADHD. [125] They are asking which neurobiological correlate links groups of symptoms in ADHD and if this correlate can be isolated from other mental functions. Authors report that in the case of individual subtypes of ADHD it could be the alteration of distinct neuronal circles. The question remains, which of these neurobiological findings explain the specific attention deficit, impulsivity, and hyperactivity as these symptoms are at the core of the ADHD-combined type. Despite the large amount of published findings about the neurobiological basis in ADHD, specific processes responsible for symptomatology of ADHD were not revealed.

Additionally, Matejcek actually mentions an evolutionary approach to ADHD which is based on the assumption that symptoms of ADHD are considered a pathological manifestation of the disorder. [168] In the past, in certain stages of development, these manifestations were considered an adaptive mechanism to living conditions. He argues whether the ADHD disorder is more of a survivor form of human adaptation than pathology.

9.3. Pharmacotherapy in ADHD

Nowadays, the symptomatology of ADHD is reduced by drugs which operate on the neurotransmitters level. The goal of treatment is to reduce the hyperactive-impulsive behavior and the attention deficit.

Bradley described children with behavioral problems who used Benzedrine and Dexedrine improved their performance at school and also had more appropriate emotional responses. [42] Bradley further states that it seems "ironic that a drug known as a stimulant could sooth behavior". [42] This paradoxical effect of stimulants became the center of pharmaceutical activities and also helped form the scientific hypothesis about the nature of ADHD. Additionally, Husarova and Ondrejka indicate that the programmed reactivity of neuronal circles is influenced by pharmaceuticals (on the level of the neurotransmitter system) and contributes to changes in post-receptor levels, thus creating an "in adequate translation" of pre-receptor information. [125] The programmed biological system has a tendency to in adequately compensate stimuli which could be an explanation for the therapy inefficiency or symptom relapse in some patients.

There are currently debates about the right choice of drugs, the length of the treatment, and the withdrawal of medication. The common practice is the withdrawal of drugs in children with ADHD on the weekends or during the summer holiday. This withdrawal can, however, lead to a gradual relapse in symptoms. The relapse of symptoms is also dependent on the length and the type of treatment. For example, Buitelaar et al. described the use of atomoxetine compared to methylphenidate was followed by a lower relapse rate. [47]

9.4. Comorbidity of ADHD

Another controversial issue in the ADHD disorder is its comorbidity. Comorbidity of a great heterogeneous spectrum of psychopathological symptoms exists in ADHD. However, the question arises whether this refer to subtypes of a single disorder with common pathomechanism or to the simultaneous occurrence of two or more disorders with different pathogenesis. [125] Given that ADHD frequently occurs with other comorbid disorders, the research needs to focus not only on finding common pathomechanism, but also on their efficacy in individual ADHD cases with the occurrence of comorbid disorders.

The very nature of the diagnosis predicts a high degree of comorbidity – symptoms and symptoms circles may or may not always occur together. Husarova and Ondrejka suggest that the actual ADHD diagnosis is comorbid *per se* and also the high degree of comorbidity in ADHD reflects the complexity of the situation. [125]

9.5. Summary

ADHD is one of the most discussed topics in terms of etiology, neurobiological correlates, pharmacotherapy, and diagnosis. A number of research efforts reflect the complexity of the disorder and at the same time are bringing more and more questions to the table. It is evident that discussions about the ADHD disorder cannot be isolated to the mental functioning of a given individual but requires interdisciplinary collaboration.

Conclusion

ADHD is a disorder that manifests itself to a greater or lesser extent in all areas of an individual life. ADHD is a disorder with exceptional variability within its etiology and manifestation. After the first efforts to define ADHD as "minimal brain damage" the scientific debate whether it is a true diagnostic category or only some specific symptoms with different etiology and associations continues to evolve into today. Efforts to categorize these symptoms into one group are problematic, and do not adequately reflect the true nature of the ailment. Current diagnostic and clinical approaches, especially the ones presented and described in the new manual of mental disorders DSM-5, show that ADHD presents the individual with major problems in individual life and their social environment. It is for the above mentioned reasons that it is necessary to address the problematic nature of ADHD and understand its variability in clinical practice and research. According to the authors of this publication, understanding the variability and how the disorder manifests itself in the real life of the sufferer is the key to its understanding. After gaining insight into the variability and the manifestation of the disorder an effective treatment strategy can be established to support to the individual.

The relatively high variability of differing viewpoints on ADHD also persists into the clinical practice. There are unconditional supporters of pharmacotherapy as the only means to treat ADHD as well as professionals who strictly oppose this type of treatment. When looking at the hundreds of available studies and especially meta-analysis that is concerned with the efficiency of the treatment it appears pharmacotherapy is the most efficient. When the proper drug is chosen pharmacotherapy can significantly improve the quality of life in children and adults with ADHD with minimal risk of side effects. Pharmacotherapy may appear to be the most efficient method of treatment but the most effective treatment was achieved when clinicians used a combined approach of pharmacotherapy and psychology. It would therefore be beneficial to seek a variable treatment solution in addressing ADHD symptom manifestations in childhood and adulthood. ADHD is, in a sense a model disorder where genetic, neurobiological, and epigenetic factors interact. ADHD is also a disorder with an exceptionally diverse range of symptoms. Therefore, great strides could be achieved in understanding the illness if ADHD became a model disorder in terms of cooperation between the fields of psychiatry, psychology, and other fields associated with it. This collaboration of the many fields would quickly create a truly effective and efficient system for treatment and would ultimately provide tremendous support to individuals with ADHD.

Despite the extraordinary advances in research about understanding the causes and mechanism of this disorder it is quite clear that it is just the beginning and much more research is required. It is highly probable that in the upcoming decades the understanding of this disorder will certainly move forward. In fact, in some of the future revisions of diagnostic classifications this disorder may be fully re-defined or linked with other diagnoses and categories. In the coming years, we can also expect a shift in the field of personalized treatment options. Existing inconsistent genetic studies show that rather than finding causative genes for this disorder it is more important to identify genetic variants that may be associated with the response to treatment.

In the future, significant advances in research and clinical practices will be prominent in the diagnosis of ADHD. The current psychological diagnostic methods were mainly created and applied for children and not to adults. The DSM-5 re-defines the ADHD diagnosis and is now requiring the need for expanded diagnostic tools for use with adolescents and adults. The current leading approach, which is based on rating and self-assessment scales, is likely to become outdated and newer more applicable objective methods of psychological diagnosis will become available. A significant shift will also happen in the area of imaging methods and their application toward a diagnosis. Despite all the hopeful advances there are still more questions than answers at the moment.

It is also expected that the current social understanding of the disorder will widen and change. In the last few decades, clinicians had to explain that children with ADHD were not "naughty" or "ill behaved" but that they were suffering from an illness were the right treatment approach could improve their behavior. Since the diagnosis of ADHD is expanding into adulthood a new level of psychoeducation in ADHD is expected to bring about understanding and lead to advances in treatment. Individuals, who are reckless, do not concentrate on work, and do not complete tasks, are not necessarily "bad people" but these individuals may be suffering from untreated ADHD symptoms that have plagued them throughout their life. The correct diagnosis and the following efficient and effective treatment can provide a major change in the sufferer in both their life and surroundings. Expanding the diagnostic criteria into other areas does, however, carry certain obvious risks. ADHD may become an excuse and a source of income for individuals and companies who will try to exploit this newly expanded diagnosis. These risks should be balanced by professional standards and by the informed approach of experts in the field of clinical medicine and its related areas.

Alternative studies suggest that ADHD is only a symptom of the modern times and it results from the accelerating pace of life and therefore is practically an inevitable phenomenon. Although these views are only speculative, they reflect the basic feature of ADHD which is its variability. Finally, through the true understanding of the variability of ADHD is where we shall find the keys to successfully diagnosing, treating, and increasing the research of this disorder.

References

[1] Acosta, M. T., Arcos-Burgos, M., & Muenke, M. (2004). Attention deficit/hyperaktivity disorder (ADHD): complex phenotype, simple genotype? *Genetics in Medicine, 6*(1), 1-15.

[2] Altafas, J. R. (2002). Prevalence of attention deficit/hyperactivity disorder among adults in obesity treatment. *BMC Psychiatry, 2*(1), 9.

[3] Amen, D. G., & Carmichael, B. D. (1997). High Resolution Brain SPECT Imaging in ADHD. *Annals of Clinical Psychiatry: Official Journal of the American Academy of Clinical Psychiatrists, 9*(2), 81–86.

[4] American Academy of Child and Adolescent Psychiatry (2002). Practice parameter for the use of stimulant medications in the treatment of children, adolescents, and adults. *Journal of the American Academy of Child and Adolescent Psychiatry, 41*(2), 26–49.

[5] American Academy of Pediatrics (2000, May). Clinical Practice Guideline: Diagnosis and Evaluation of the Child with Attention-Deficit/Hyperactivity Disorder. Committee on Quality Improvement, Subcommittee on Attention-Deficit/Hyperactivity Disorder. *Pediatrics, 105*(5), 1158-1170.

[6] American Psychiatric Association (1952). *Diagnostic and Statistic manual of mental disorders, 1st ed.* Washington DC: American Psychiatric Association.

[7] American Psychiatric Association (1968). *Diagnostic and Statistic manual of mental disorders, 2nd ed.* Washington DC: American Psychiatric Association.

[8] American Psychiatric Association (1980). *Diagnostic and Statistic manual of mental disorders, 3rd ed.* Washington DC: American Psychiatric Association.

[9] American Psychiatric Association (1987). *Diagnostic and Statistic manual of mental disorders, 3rd ed. revised.* Washington DC: American psychiatric Association.

[10] American Psychiatric Association (1994). *Diagnostic and Statistic manual of mental disorders, 4th ed.* Washington DC: American psychiatric Association.

[11] American Psychiatric Association (2000). *Diagnostic and Statistic manual of mental disorders, 4th ed. text rev.* Washington DC: American psychiatric Association.

[12] American Psychiatric Association (2013). *Diagnostic and Statistic manual of mental disorders, 5th ed.* Washington DC: American psychiatric Association.

[13] Andrews, G. D., & Lavin, A. (2006). Methylphenidate increases cortical excitability via activation of alpha-2 noradrenergic receptors. *Neuropsychopharmacology, 31*(3), 594–601.

[14] Arcos-Burgos, M., Castellanos, F. X., Pineda, D., Lopera, F., Palacio, J. D., Palacio, L. G., et al. (2004). Attention-deficit/hyperactivity disorder in a population isolate: linkage to loci at 4q13.2, 5q33.3, 11q22, and 17p11. *The American Journal of Human Genetics, 75*(6), 998–1014.

[15] Arnold, L. E. (1996, October). Sex differences in ADHD: conference summary. *Journal of Abnormal Child Psychology, 24*(5), 555-569.

[16] Asherson, P., Zhou, K., Anney, R. J., Franke, B., Buitelaar, J., Ebstein, R., et al. (2008). A high-density SNP linkage scan with 142 combined subtype ADHD sib pairs identifies linkage regions on chromosomes 9 and 16. *Molecular Psychiatry, 13*(5), 514–521.

[17] Ayres, A. J. (2005). *Sensory integration and the child, 25th anniversary edition*. Los Angeles: Western Psychological Services.

[18] Bakker, S. C., van der Meulen, E. M., Buitelaar, J. K., Sandkuijl, L. A., Pauls, D. L., Monsuur, A. J., et al. (2003). A whole-genome scan in 164 Dutch sib pairs with attentiondeficit/ hyperactivity disorder: suggestive evidence for linkage on chromosomes 7p and 15q. *The American Journal of Human Genetics, 72*(5), 1251–1260.

[19] Banaschewski, T., Coghill, D., Santosh, P., Zuddas, A., Asherson, P., Buitelaar, J., et al. (2006). Long-acting medications for the hyperkinetic disorders. A systematic review and European treatment guideline. *European Child & Adolescent Psychiatry, 15*(8), 476–495.

[20] Banerjee, T. D., Middleton, F., & Faraone, S. V. (2007). Environmental risk factors for attention-deficit hyperactivity disorder. *Acta Paediatrica, 96*(9), 1269-1274.

[21] Barkley, R. A. (1990). *Attention-Deficit Hyperactivity Disorder: A Handbook for Diagnosis and Treatment.* New York: Guilford Press.

[22] Barkley, R. A. (1997). *Defiant children: A clinician´s manual for parent training*. New York: Guilford Press.

[23] Barkley, R. A. (2006). *Attention deficit hyperactivity disorder: A Handbook for diagnosis and treatment.* New York: Guilford Press.

[24] Barkley, R. A., & Macias, M. (2005). Attention deficit hyperactivity disorder. In R. David (Ed.), *Child and adolescent neurology (3rd ed.).* New York: Blackwell.

[25] Barzman, D. H., Patel, A., Sonnier, L., & Strawn, J. R. (2010). Neuroendocrine aspects of pediatric aggression: Can hormone measures be clinically useful? *Neuropsychiatric Disease and Treatment, 6*, 691-697.

[26] Bazar, K. A., Yun, A. J., Lee, P. Y., Daniel, S. M., & Doux, J. D. (2006). Obesity and ADHD may represent different manifestations of a common environmental oversampling syndrome: a model for revealing mechanistic overlap among cognitive, metabolic, and inflammatory disorders. *Medical Hypotheses 66*(2), 263-269.

[27] Becker, K., Buitelaar, J. K., Danckaerts, M., Gillberg, C., Zuddas, A., Bouvard, M., et al. (2004). Does atomoxetine treatment improve psychosocial and family functioning in children and adolescents with ADHD? *Acta Psychiatrica Scandinavica, 110*(421), 48-49.

[28] Bedard, A. C. V., Trampush, J. W., Newcorn, J. H., & Halperin, J. H. (2010). Perceptual and Motor Inhibition in Adolescents/Young Adults with Childhood-Diagnosed ADHD. *Neuropsychology, 24*(4), 424–434.

[29] Beitchman, J. H., Nair, R., Clegg, M., Ferguson, B., & Patel, P. G. (1986). Prevalence of psychiatric disorders in children with speech and language disorders. *Journal of the American Academy of Child Psychiatry, 25*(4), 528-535.

[30] Bhaduri, N., Sarkar, K., Sinha, S., Chattopadhyay, A., & Mukhopadhyay, K. (2010, March). Study on DBH genetic polymorphisms and plasma activity in attention deficit hyperactivity disorder patients from Eastern India. *Cellular and Molecular Neurobiology, 30*(2), 265-274.

[31] Biederman, J., & Spencer, T. J. (2008). Psychopharmacological interventions. *Child and Adolescent Psychiatric Clinic of North America, 17*(2), 439-458.

[32] Biederman, J., Ball, S. W., Monuteaux, M. C., Surman, C. B., Johnson, J. L., & Zeitlin, S. (2007, August). Are girls with ADHD at risk for

eating disorders? Results from a controlled, five-year prospective study. *Journal of Developmental and Behavioral Pediatrics, 28*(4), 302-307.

[33] Biederman, J., Faraone, S. V., Keenan, K., Knee, D., & Tsuang, M. T. (1990). Family-genetic and psychosocial risk factors in DSM-III attention deficit disorder. *Journal of the American Academy of Child and Adolescent Psychiatry, 29*(4), 526–533.

[34] Biederman, J., Faraone, S. V., Keenan, K., & Tsuang, M. T. (1991, July). Evidence of familial association between attention deficit disorder and major affective disorders. *Archives of General Psychiatry. 48*(7), 633-642.

[35] Biederman, J., Faraone, S. V., Monuteaux, M. C., Plunkett, E. A., Gifford, J., & Spencer, T. (2003a). Growth deficits and attention-deficit/hyperactivity disorder revisited: impact of gender, development and treat-ment. *Pediatrics, 111*(1), 1010–1016.

[36] Biederman, J., Mick, E., Wozniak, J., Monuteaux, M. C., Galdo, M., & Faraone, S. V. (2003b). Can a subtype of conduct disorder linked to bipolar disorder be identified? Integration of findings from the Massachusetts General Hospital Pediatric Psychopharmacology Research Program. *Biological Psychiatry, 53*(11), 952-960.

[37] Biederman, J., Spencer, T. J., Monuteaux, M. C., & Faraone, S. V. (2010, October). A naturalistic 10-year prospective study of height and weight in children with attention-deficit hyperactivity disorder grown up: sex and treatment effects. *Journal of Pediatrics, 157*(4), 635-640.

[38] Blinder, B. J., Cumella, E. J., & Sanathara, V. A. (2006). Psychiatric comorbidities of female inpatients with eating disorders. *Psychosomatic Medicine, 68*(3), 454-462.

[39] Blom, R. M., Samuels, J. F., Riddle, M. A., Joseph Bienvenu, O., Grados, M. A., Reti, I. M., et al. (2011, September). Association between a serotonin transporter promoter polymorphism (5HTTLPR) and personality disorder traits in a community sample. *Journal of Psychiatric Research, 45*(9), 1153-1159.

[40] Bobb, A. J., Addington, A. M., Sidransky, E., Gornick, M. C., Lerch, J. P., Greenstein, D. K., et al. (2005). Support for association between ADHD and two candidate genes: NET1 and DRD1. *American Journal of Medical Geneticst Part B, Neuropsychiatric Genetics, 134*(1), 67–72.

[41] Bradley, C. (1937). The behavior of children receiving benzedrine. *The American Journal of Psychiatry, 94*(3), 577-585.

[42] Bradley, C. (1950). Benzedrine and dexedrine in the treatment of children's behavior disorders. *Pediatrics, 5*(1), 24-36.

[43] Brophy, K., Hawi, Z., Kirley, A., Fitzgerald, M., & Gill, M. (2002). Synaptosomal-associated protein 25 (SNAP-25) and attention deficit hyperactivity disorder (ADHD): evidence of linkage and association in the Irish population. *Molecular Psychiatry, 7*(8), 913-917.

[44] Brown, R. T., Amler, R. W., Freeman, W. S., Perrin, J. M., Stein, J. M., Feldman, H. M., et al. (2005). Treatment of Attention-Deficit/Hyperactivity Disorder: Overview of the Evidence. *Pediatrics, 115*(6), 749-757.

[45] Buderath, P., Gartner, K., Frings, M., Christiansen, H., Schoch, B., Konczak, J., et al. (2009). Postural and gait performance in children with attention deficit/hyperaktivity disorder. *Gait & Posture, 29*(2), 249-254.

[46] Budziszewska, B., Basta-Kaim, A., Kubera, M., & Lasoń, W. (2010). Immunological and endocrinological pattern in ADHD etiopathogenesis. *Przeglad Lekarski, 67*(11), 1200-1204.

[47] Buitelaar, J., Michelson, D., Danckaerts, M., Gillberg, C., Spencer, T. J., Zuddas, A., et al. (2007, March). A randomized, double-blind study of continuation treatment for attention-deficit/hyperactivity disorder after 1 year. *Biological Psychiatry, 61*(5), 694-699.

[48] Busch, B. (2007, April). Polyunsaturated fatty acid supplementation for ADHD? Fishy, fascinating, and far from clear. *Journal of Developmental and Behavioral Pediatrics, 28*(2), 139-144.

[49] Bush, G., Frazier, J. A., Rauch, S. L., Seidman, L. J., Whalen, P. J., Jenike, M. A., et al. (1999). Anterior cingulate cortex dysfunction in attention-deficit/hyperactivity disorder revealed by fMRI and the Counting Stroop. *Biological Psychiatry, 45*(12), 1542-1552.

[50] Buzy, W. M., Medoff, D. R., & Schweitzer, J. B. (2009, September). Intraindividual variability among children with ADHD on a working memory task: an ex-gaussian approach. *Child Neuropsychology, 15*(5), 441–459.

[51] Cahova, P., Pejcochova, J., & Oslejskova, H. (2010). Hyperkineticka porucha/ADHD v dospivani a dospelosti: diagnostika, klinicky obraz a komorbidity. *Neurologie pro praxi, 11*(6), 367–371.

[52] Cardinal, R. N., Pennicott, D. R., Sugathapala, C. L., Robbins, T. W., & Everitt, B. J. (2001). Impulsive choice induced in rats by lesions of the nucleus accumbens core. *Science, 292*(5526), 2499–2500.

[53] Castel, A. D., Lee, S. S., Humphreys, K. L., & Moore, A. N. (2011, January). Memory capacity, selective control, and value-directed

remembering in children with and without attention-deficit/hyperactivity disorder (ADHD). *Neuropsychology, 25*(1), 15-24.

[54] Castellanos, F. X., Lee, P. P., Sharp, W., Jeffries, N. O., Greenstein, D. K., Clasen, L. S., et al. (2002). Developmental trajectories of brain volume abnormalities in children and adolescents with attention-deficit/hyperactivity disorder. *The Journal of American Medical Association, 288*(14), 1740-1748.

[55] Charach, A., Figueroa, M., Chen, S., Ickowicz, A., & Schachar, R. (2006). Stimulant Treatment Over 5 Years: Effects on Growth. *Journal of the American Academy of Child and Adolescent Psychiatry, 45*(4), 415-421.

[56] Charach, A., Ickowicz, A., & Schachar, R. (2004, May). Stimulant treatment over five years: adherence, effectiveness, and adverse effects. *Journal of the American Academy of Child and Adolescent Psychiatry, 43*(5), 559-567.

[57] Cheon, K. A., Ryu, Y. H., Kim, J. W., & Cho, D. Y. (2005, January). The homozygosity for 10-repeat allele at dopamine transporter gene and dopamine transporter density in Korean children with attention deficit hyperactivity disorder: relating to treatment response to methylphenidate. *European Neuropsychopharmacology, 15*(1), 95-101.

[58] Chess, S. (1960, August). Diagnosis and treatment of the hyperactive child. *New York State Journal of Medicine, 60*, 2379-2385.

[59] Clarke, A. R., Barry, R. J., McCarthy, R., Selikowitz, M., Clarke, D. C., & Croft, R. J. (2003, February). EEG activity in girls with attention-deficit/hyperactivity disorder. *Clinical Neurophysiology, 114*(2), 319-328.

[60] Coghill, D. R., Rhodes, S. M., & Matthews, K. (2007). The neuropsychological effects of chronic methylphenidate on drug-naive boys with attention-deficit/ hyperactivity disorder. *Biological Psychiatry, 62*(9), 954-962.

[61] Cohen, N. J., Vallance, D. D., Barwick, M., Im, N., Menna, R., Horodezky, N. B, et al. (2000, March). The interface between ADHD and language impairment: an examination of language, achievement, and cognitive processing. *Journal of Child Psychology and Psychiatry, 41*(3), 353-362.

[62] Conners, C. K. (2008). *Conners 3rd edition. Manual.* New York: Multi-Health System.

[63] Conners, C. K., & Multi-Health Systems Staff. (Eds.) (2000). *Conners' Continuous Performance Test II: Computer Program for Windows*

Technical Guide and Software Manual. North Tonawanda: Multi-Health Systems.

[64] Conners, C. K., Wells, K. C., Parker, J. D., Sitarenios, G., Diamond, J. M., & Powell, J. W. (1997, December). A new self-report scale for assessment of adolescent psychopathology: factor structure, reliability, validity, and diagnostic sensitivity. *Journal of Abnormal Child Psychology, 25*(6), 487-497.

[65] Coolidge, F. L., Thede, L. L., & Young, S. E. (2000). Heritability and the comorbidity of attention deficit hyperactivity disorder with behavioral disorders and executive function deficits: a preliminary investigation. *Developmental Neuropsychology, 17*(3), 273–287.

[66] Cortese, S., Angriman, M., Maffeis, C., Isnard, P., Konofal, E., Lecendreux, M., et al. (2008, September). Attention-deficit/hyperactivity disorder (ADHD) and obesity: a systematic review of the literature. *Critical Reviews in Food Science and Nutrition, 48*(6), 524-537.

[67] Cortese, S., Bernardina, B. D., & Mouren, M. C. (2007, September). Attention-deficit/hyperactivity disorder (ADHD) and binge eating. *Nutrition Reviews, 65*(9), 404-411.

[68] Cruz, N. V., & Bahna, S. L. (2006). Do food or additives cause behavior disorders? *Pediatric Annals, 35*(10), 748-754.

[69] Cubillo, A., Halari, R., Smith, A., Taylor, E., & Rubia, K. (2012, February). A review of fronto-striatal and fronto-cortical brain abnormalities in children and adults with Attention Deficit Hyperactivity Disorder (ADHD) and new evidence for dysfunction in adults with ADHD during motivation and attention. *Cortex, 48*(2), 194-215.

[70] Curatolo, P., D'Agati, E., & Moavero, R. (2010). The neurobiological basis of ADHD. *Italian Journal of Pediatrics, 36*(1), 79-85.

[71] Curtin, C., Bandini, L. G., Perrin, E. C., Tybor, D. J., & Must, A. (2005). Prevalence of overweight in children and adolescents with attention deficit hyperactivity disorder and autism spectrum disorders: a chart review. *BioMed Central Pediatrics, 5*(1), 48-58.

[72] D'Agati, E., Casarelli, L., Pitzianti, M. B., & Pasini, A. (2010). Overflow movements and white matter abnormalities in ADHD. *Progress in Neuropsychopharmacology and Biological Psychiatry, 34*(3), 441-445.

[73] Da Silva, T. L., Pianca, T. G., Roman, T., Hutz, H. M., Faraone, S. V., Schmitz, M., et al. (2008). Adrenergic alpha2A receptor gene and

response to methylphenidate in attention-deficit/hyperactivity disorder-predominantly inattentive type. *Journal of Neural Transmission, 115*(2), 341-345.

[74] Daly, G., Hawi, Z., Fitzgerald, M., & Gill, M. (1999). Mapping susceptibility loci in attention deficit hyperactivity disorder: preferential transmission of parentel alleles at DAT1, DBH and DRD5 to affected children. *Molecular Psychiatry, 4*(2), 192–196.

[75] Davis, C., & Carter, J. C. (2009, August). Compulsive overeating as an addiction disorder. A review of theory and evidence. *Appetite, 53*(1), 1-8.

[76] Davis, C., Levitan, R. D., Kaplan, A. S., Carter, J., Reid, C., Curtis, C., et al. (2008). Reward sensitivity and the D2 receptor gene: a case-control study of binge eating disorder. *Progress in Neuro-Psychopharmacology and Biological Psychiatry, 32*(3), 620-628.

[77] Doggett, A. M. (2004, March). ADHD and drug therapy: is it still a valid treatment? *Journal of Child Health Care, 8*(1), 69-81.

[78] Donahoo, W., Wyatt, H. R., Kriehn, J., Stuht, J., Dong, F., Hosokawa, P., et al. (2008, January). Dietary fat increases energy intake across the range of typical consumption in the United States. *Obesity (Silver Spring), 16*(1), 64-69.

[79] Drappatz, J., Khwaja, O. S., Neovius, M., & Sarco, D. S. (2006). Growth in Children with ADHD Treated with Stimulant Medications: A Meta-Analysis. *Pediatric Academic Societies Annual Meeting, 3*, 458.

[80] Drtilova, J., & Koukolnik, F. (1994). *Odlisne dite.* Praha: Vysehrad.

[81] Drtilkova, I. (2003). Ucinnost nestandardnich postupu lecby u deti s ADHD. *Ceska a slovenska Psychiatrie, 99*(6),317-323.

[82] Drtilkova, I. (2007). *Hyperaktivni dite: Vse, co potrebujete vedet o diteti s hyperkinetickou poruchou (ADHD).* Praha: Galen.

[83] Drtilkova, I. (2008). Soucasny pohled na hyperkinetickou poruchu/ADHD a nove moznosti jeji lecby. *Lekarske listy, 16*, 8.

[84] Drtilkova, I., & Sery, O. (2007). *Hyperkineticky syndrom.* Praha: Galen.

[85] Drtilkova, I., Hrdlicka, M., & Paclt, I. (2006). Hyperkineticke poruchy u deti. In J. Raboch, M. Anders, J. Prasko & P. Hellerova (Eds.), *Psychiatrie: Doporucene postupy psychiatricke pece II.* (pp. 141-149). Praha: Ceska lekarska spolecnost Jana Evangelisty Purkyne.

[86] Dudova, I., & Hrdlicka, M. (2003). Hyperkineticke poruchy v detstvi. *Postgradualni medicina, 7.*

[87] Durston, S., Fossella, J. A., Casey, B. J., Hulshoff Pol, H. E., Galvan, A., Schnack, H. G., et al. (2005). Differential effects of DRD4 and

DAT1 genotype on fronto-striatal gray matter volumes in a sample of subjects with attention deficit hyperactivity disorder, their unaffected siblings, and controls. *Molecular Psychiatry, 10*(7), 678–685.

[88] Eiraldi, R. B., Mazzuca, L. B., Clarke, A. T., & Power, T. J. (2006, September). Service Utilization among ethnic minority children with ADHD: a model of help-seeking behavior. *Administration and Policy in Mental Health, 33*(5), 607-622.

[89] Ellison-Wright, I., Ellison-Wright, Z., & Bullmore, E. (2008, June). Structural brain change in Attention Deficit Hyperactivity Disorder identified by meta-analysis. *BioMed Central Psychiatry, 8*(1), 51-58.

[90] Emond, V., Joyal, C., & Poissant, H. (2009). Structural and functional neuroanatomy of attention-deficit hyperactivity disorder (ADHD). *Encephale, 35*(2), 107-114.

[91] Faraone, S. V. (2009b). Using Meta-analysis to Compare the Efficacy of Medications for Attention-Deficit/Hyperactivity Disorder in Youths. *Physical Therapy, 34*(12), 678-694.

[92] Faraone, S. V., & Giefer, E. E. (2007). Long-Term Effects of Methylphenidate Transdermal Delivery System Treatment of ADHD on Growth. *Journal of the American Academy of Child Adolescent Psychiatry, 46*(9), 1138-1147.

[93] Faraone, S. V., & Mick, E. (2010). Molecular genetics of attention deficit hyperactivity disorder. *Psychiatric Clinics of North America, 33*(1), 159-180.

[94] Faraone, S. V., Biederman, J., Morley, C. P., & Spencer, T. J. (2008, September). Effect of stimulants on height and weight: a review of the literature. *Journal of the American Academy of Child and Adolesccent Psychiatry, 47*(9), 994–1009.

[95] Faraone, S. V., Perlis, R. H., Doyle, A. E., Smoller, J. W., Goralnick, J. J., Holmogren, M. A., et al. (2005). Molecular genetics of attention deficit hyperactivity disorder. *Biological Psychiatry, 57*(11), 1313-1323.

[96] Faraone, S. V., Pucci, M., & Coghill, D. (2009a, April). Pharmacotherapy for Attention-deficit Hyperactivity disorder. *European Psychiatry Review, 2*(1), 42-52.

[97] Fassbender, C., Schweitzer, J. B., Cortes, C. R., Tagamets, M. A., Windsor, T. A., Reeves, G. M., et al. (2011, November). Working memory in attention deficit/hyperactivity disorder is characterized by a lack of specialization of brain function. *Public Library of Science, 6*(11), 1-11.

[98] Fisher, S. E., Francks, C., McCracken, J. T., McGough, J. J., Marlow, A. J., MacPhie, I. L., et al. (2002). A genomewide scan for loci involved in attention-deficit/hyperactivity disorder. *American Journal of Human Genetics, 70*(5), 1183–1196.

[99] Fliers, E., Rommelse, N., Vermeulen, S. H., Altink, M., Buschgens, C. J., Faraone, S. V., et al. (2008). Motor coordination problems in children and adolescents with ADHD rated by parents and teachers: effects of age and gender. *Journal of Neural Transmission, 115*(2), 211-220.

[100] Franke, B., Neale, B. M., & Faraone, S. V. (2009b). Genome-wide association studies in ADHD. *Human Genetics, 126*(1), 13-50.

[101] Franke, B., Vasquez, A. A., Johansson, S., Hoogman, M., Romanos, J., Boreatti-Hummer, A., et al. (2009a). Multicenter Analysis of the SLC6A3/DAT1 VNTR Haplotype in Persistent ADHD Suggests Differential Involvement of the Gene in Childhood and Persistent ADHD. *Neuropsychopharmacology, 35*(3), 656-664.

[102] Freitag, C. M., Hänig, S., Palmason, H., Meyer, J., Wüst, S., & Seitz, C. (2009, August). Cortisol awakening response in healthy children and children with ADHD: impact of comorbid disorders and psychosocial risk factors. *Psychoneuroendocrinology, 34*(7), 1019-1028.

[103] Frindik, J. P., Fowlkes, J., Kemp, S. F., Thrailkill, K., Morales, A., & Dana, K. (2009). Stimulant Medication Use and Response to Growth Hormone Therapy: An NCGS Database Analysis. *Hormone Research, 72*(3), 160–166.

[104] Fusar-Poli, P., Rubia, K., Rossi, G., Sartori, G., & Balottin, U. (2012, March). Striatal dopamine transporter alterations in ADHD: pathophysiology or adaptation to psychostimulants? A meta-analysis. *American Journal of Psychiatry, 169*(3), 264-272.

[105] Gesell, A., & Amatruda, C. S. (1947). *Developmental diagnosis (2nd ed.).* New York: Hoeber Publishing Co.

[106] Gilger, J. W., Pennington, B. F., & DeFries, J. C. (1992). A twin study of the etiology of comorbidity: attention-deficit hyperactivity disorder and dyslexia. *Journal of the American Academy of Child and Adolescent Psychiatry, 31*(2), 343-348.

[107] Gizer, I. R., Ficks, C., & Waldman, I. D. (2009). Candidate gene studies of ADHD: a metaanalytic review. *Human Genetics, 126*(1), 51-90.

[108] Goetz, M. (2006). ADHD u dospelych. *Postgradualni medicina, 3*, 270-276.

[109] Goetz, M., & Uhlikova, P. (2009). *ADHD Porucha pozornosti s hyperaktivitou.* Praha: Galen.

[110] Goodman, D. W., & Thase, M. E. (2009). Recognizing ADHD in Adults with Comorbid Mood Disorders: Implications for Identification and Management. *Postgraduate Medicine, 121*(5), 1-11.

[111] Gremillion, M. L., & Martel, M. M. (2012). Semantic Language as a Mechanism Explaining the Association between ADHD Symptoms and Reading and Mathematics Underachievement. *Journal of Abnormal Child Psychology, 40*(8), 1339-1349.

[112] Guerrieri, R., Nederkoorn, C., & Jansen, A. (2008). The interaction between impulsivity and a varied food environment: its influence on food intake and overweight. *International Journal of Obesity, 32*(4), 708–714.

[113] Guerrieri, R., Nederkoorn, C., Schrooten, M., Martijn, C., & Jansen, A. (2009, August). Inducing impulsivity leads high and low restrained eaters into overeating, whereas current dieters stick to their diet. *Appetite, 53*(1), 93-100.

[114] Hallowell, E. M., & Ratey, J. J. (1995). *Driven to Distraction: Recognizing and Coping with Attention Deficit Disorder from Childhood Through Adulthood.* New York: Times Review.

[115] Hamarman, S., Fossella, J., Ulger, C., Brimacombe, M., & Dermody, J. (2004). Dopamine receptor 4 (DRD4) 7-repeat allele predicts methylphenidate dose response in children with attention deficit hyperactivity disorder: a pharmacogenetic study. *Journal of Child and Adolescent Psychopharmacology, 14*(4), 564-574.

[116] Hastings, P. D., Fortier, I., Utendale, W. T., Simard, L. R., & Robaey, P. (2009, May). Adrenocortical functioning in boys with attention-deficit/hyperactivity disorder: examining subtypes of ADHD and associated comorbid conditions. *Journal of Abnormal Child Psychology, 37*(4), 565-578.

[117] Hatzinger, M., Brand, S., Perren, S., von Wyl, A., von Klitzing, K., & Holsboer-Trachsler, E. (2007, November). Hypothalamic - pituitary - adrenocortical (HPA) activity in kindergarten children: importance of gender and associations with behavioral/emotional difficulties. *Journal Psychiatr Research, 41*(10), 861-870.

[118] Hauser, P., Soler, R., Brucker-Davis, F., & Weintraub, B. D. (1997, February). Thyroid hormones correlate with symptoms of hyperactivity but not inattention in attention deficit hyperactivity disorder. *Psychoneuroendocrinology, 22*(2), 107-114.

[119] Hebebrand, J., Dempfle, A., Saar, K., Thiele, H., Herpertz-Dahlmann, B., Linder, M., et al. (2006). A genomewide scan for attention-

deficit/hyperactivity disorder in 155 German sib-pairs. *Molecular Psychiatry, 11*(2), 196–205.

[120] Heinz, A., & Smolka, M. N. (2006). The effects of catechol O-methyltransferase genotype on brain activation elicited by affective stimuli and cognitive tasks. *Annual Review of Neuroscience, 17*(3), 359-367.

[121] Holtkamp, K., Konrad, K., Müller, B., Heussen, N., Herpertz, S., Herpertz-Dahlmann, B., et al. (2004, May). Overweight and obesity in children with Attention-Deficit/Hyperactivity Disorder. *International Journal of Obesity and Related Metabolic Disorders, 28*(5), 685-689.

[122] Hort, V., Hrdlička, M., Kocourková, J., & Malá, E. (2000). *Dětská a adolescentní psychiatrie.* Praha: Portál.

[123] Hrdlicka, M. (2007). Postaveni atomoxetinu v lecbe hyperkineticke poruchy u deti a adolescentu. *Ceska a slovenska Psychiatrie, 103*(5), 230-239.

[124] Hubel, R., Jass, J., Marcus, A., & Laessle, R. G. (2006, September). Overweight and basal metabolic rate in boys with attention-deficit/hyperactivity disorder. *Eating and Weight Disorders, 11*(3), 139-146.

[125] Husarova, V., & Ondrejka, I. (2012). ADHD: Stale veľa otazok. *Ceska a slovenska Psychiatria, 108*(3), 131-137.

[126] Iseri, E., Kilic, B. G., Senol, S., & Karabacak, N. I. (2007, January-February). Effects of methylphenidate on leptin and appetite in children with attention-deficit hyperactivity disorder: an open label trial. *Methods and Findings in Experimental and Clinical Pharmacology, 29*(1), 47-52.

[127] Itoi. K, & Sugimoto, N. (2010, May). The brainstem noradrenergic systems in stress, anxiety and depression. *Journal of Neuroendocrinology, 22*(5), 355-361.

[128] Jensen, P. S., Hinshaw, S. P., Kraemer, H. C., Lenora, N., Newcorn, J. H., Abikoff, H. B., et al. (2001, February). ADHD comorbidity findings from the MTA study: comparing comorbid subgroups. *Journal of the American Academy of Child and Adolescent Psychiatry, 40*(2), 147-158.

[129] Jiang, S. D., He, M., Qian, Y. P., Wang, D. X., Zhang, Y., Li, F., et al. (2006). Genome-wide search for linkage to attention deficit hyperactivity disorder (ADHD) on the X chromosome. *Yi Chuan, 28*(1), 26–30.

[130] Joober, R., Grizenko, N., Sengupta, S., Amor, L. B., Schmitz, N., Schwartz, G., et al. (2007, June). Dopamine transporter 30-UTR VNTR

genotype and ADHD: a pharmaco-behavioural genetic study with methylphenidate. *Neuropsychopharmacology, 32*(6), 1370-1376.

[131] Joseph, J. (2000). Not in Their Genes: A Critical View of the Genetics of Attention-Deficit Hyperactivity Disorder. *Developmental Review 20*(4), 539–567.

[132] Kalachnik, J. E., Sprague, R. L., Sleator, E. K., Cohen, M. N., & Ullmann, R. K. (1982). Effect of methylphenidate hydrochloride on stature of hyperactive children. *Developmental Medicine and Child Neurology, 24*(5), 586–595.

[133] Karatekin, C., Markiewicz, S. W., & Siegel, M. A. (2003). A preliminary study of motor problems in children with attention-Deficit/Hyperactivity disorder. *Perceptual and Motor Skills, 97*(2), 1267-1280.

[134] Kereszturi, E., Tarnok, Z., Bognar, E., Lakatos, K., Farkas, L., Gadoros, J., et al. (2008, January). Catechol-Omethyltransferase Val158Met polymorphism is associated with methylphenidate response in ADHD children. *American Journal of Medical Genetics Part B, Neuropsychiatric Genetics, 147*(8), 1431-1435.

[135] Kessler, R. C., Adler, L., Barkley, R., Biederman, J., Conners, C. K., Demler, O., et al. (2006, April). The prevalence and correlates of adult ADHD in the United States: results from the National Comorbidity Survey Replication. *American Journal of Psychiatry, 163*(4), 716-723.

[136] Kessler, R. C., Green, J. G., Adler, L. A., Barkley, R. A., Chatterji, S., Faraone, S. V., et al. (2010, November). Structure and diagnosis of adult attention-deficit/hyperactivity disorder: analysis of expanded symptom criteria from the Adult ADHD Clinical Diagnostic Scale. *Archives of General Psychiatry, 67*(11), 1168-1178.

[137] Kim, J. W., Biederman, J., Arbeitman, L., Fagerness, J., Doyle, A. E., Petty, C., et al. (2007, September). Investigation of variation in SNAP-25 and ADHD and relationship to co-morbid major depressive disorder. *American Journal of Medical Genetics Part B, Neuropsychiatric Genetics*, *144*(6), 781-790.

[138] King, J. A., Barkley, R. A., & Barrett, S. (1998). Attention-Deficit Hyperactivity Disorder and the Stress Response. *Journal of Biological Psychiatry, 44*(1), 73-74.

[139] Klein, R. G., Landa, B., Mattes, J. A., & Klein, D. F. (1988). Methylphenidate and growth in hyperactive children. A control-led withdrawal study. *Archives of General Psychiatry, 45*(12), 1127–1130.

[140] Klimkeit, E. I., Sheppard, D. M., Lee, P., & Bradshaw, J. L. (2004). Bimanual coordination deficits in attention Deficit/Hyperactivity disorder (ADHD). *Journal of Clinical and Experimental Neuropsychology, 26*(8), 999-1010.

[141] Knouse, L. E., Cooper-Vince, C., Sprich, S., & Safren, S. (2008, October). Recent developments in the psychosocial treatment of adult ADHD. *Expert Review of Neurotherapeutics, 8*(10), 1537–1548.

[142] Kooistra, L., Crawford, S., Dewey, D., Cantell, M., & Kaplan, B. J. (2005, May-June). Motor correlates of ADHD: contribution of reading disability and oppositional defiant disorder. *Journal of Learning Disabilities, 38*(3), 195-206.

[143] Kopeckova, M., Paclt, I., Petrasek, J., Pacltova, D., Malikova, M., & Zagatova, V. (2008, April). Some ADHD polymorphisms (in genes DAT1, DRD2, DRD3, DBH, 5-HTT) in case-control study of 100 subjects 6-10 age. *Neuro Endocrinology Letters, 29*(2), 246-251.

[144] Kotimaa, A. J., Moilanen, I., Taanila, A., Ebeling, H., Smalley, S. L., McGough, J. J., et al. (2003, July). Maternal smoking and hyperactivity in 8-year-old children. *Journal of the American Acadeny of Child and Adolescent Psychiatry, 42*(7), 826-833.

[145] Kovacs-Nagy, R., Hu, J., Ronai, Z., & Sasvari-Szekely, M. (2009, June). SNAP-25: a novel candidate gene in psychiatric genetics. *Neuropsychopharmacol Hung, 11*(2), 89-94.

[146] Krain, A. L., & Castellanos, F. X. (2006). Brain development and ADHD. *Clinical Psychology Review, 26*(4), 433-444.

[147] Kratochvil, C. J., Egger, H., Greenhill, L. L., & McGough, J. J. (2006a). Pharmacological management of preschool ADHD. *Journal of the American Academy of Child and Adolescent Psychiatry, 45*(1), 115–118.

[148] Kratochvil, C. J., Milton, D. R., Vaughan, B. S., & Greenhill, L. L. (2008). Acute atomoxetine treatment of younger and older children with ADHD: a meta-analysis of tolerability and efficacy. *Child and Adolescent Psychiatry and Mental Health, 2*(1), 25.

[149] Kratochvil, C. J., Wilens, T. E., Greenhill, L. L., Gao, H., Baker, K. D., Feldman, P. D., et al. (2006b). Effects of long-term atomoxetine treatment for young children with attention-deficit/hyperactivity disorder. *Journal of the American Academy of Child and Adolescent Psychiatry, 45*(8), 919-927.

[150] Kreppner, J. M., O'Connor, T. G., & Rutter, M. (2001, December). English and Romanian Adoptees Study Team. Can

inattention/overactivity be an institutional deprivation syndrome? *Journal of Abnormal Child Psychology, 29*(6), 513-528.

[151] Kuzelova, H., Ptacek, R., & Macek, M. (2010). The serotonin transporter gene (5-HTT) variant and psychiatric disorders: review of current literature. *Neuro Endocrinology Letters, 31*(1), 4-10.

[152] Laakso, A., Pohjalainen, T., Bergman, J., Kajander, J., Haaparanta, M., Solin, O., et al. (2005). The Al allele of the human D2 dopamine receptor gene is associated with increased activity of striatal L-amino acid decarboxylase in healthy subjects. *Pharmacogenetics and Genomics, 15*(6), 387-391.

[153] Lam, L. T., & Yang, L. (2007). Overweight/obesity and attention deficit and hyperactivity disorder tendency among adolescents in China. *International Journal of Obesity, 31*(4), 584-590.

[154] Lambert, N. M., & Hartsough, C. S. (1998, November-December). Prospective study of tobacco smoking and substance dependencies among samples of ADHD and non-ADHD participants. *Journal of Learning Disabilities, 31*(6), 533-544.

[155] Laufer, M. W., Denhoff, E., & Solomons, G. (1957). Hyperactive Impulsive Disorder in Children's Behaviour Problems. *Psychosomatic Medicine, 19*, 38-49.

[156] Levy, F. (2009, February). Dopamine vs noradrenaline: inverted-U effects and ADHD theories. *Australian and New Zealand Journal of Psychiatry, 43*(2), 101-108.

[157] Lezak, M. D. (2004). *Neuropsychological assessment.* New York: Oxford Univerzity Press.

[158] Li, J., Wang, Y., Zhou, R., Zhang, H., Yang, L., Wang, B., et al. (2006). Association between tryptophan hydroxylase gene polymorphisms and attention deficit hyperactivity disorder in Chinese Han population. *American Journal of Medical Genetics Part B, Neuropsychiatric Genetics, 141*(2), 126–129.

[159] Liebson, C. L., Katusic, S. K., Barbaresi, W. J., Ransom, J., & O´Brien, P. C. (2001, January). Use and costs of medical care for children and adolescents with and without attention-deficit/hyperactivity disorder. *Journal of the American Medical Association, 285*(1), 60-66.

[160] Lisska, M. C., & Rivkees, S. A. (2003). Daily methylphenidate use slows the growth of children: a community based study. *Journal of Pediatric Endocrinology Metabolism, 16*(5), 711-718.

[161] Luders, E., Narr, K. L., Hamilton, L. S., Phillips, O. R., Thompson, P. M., Valle, J. S., et al. (2009). Decreased callosal thickness in attention-deficit/hyperactivity disorder. *Biological Psychiatry, 65*(1), 84-88.

[162] Ma, L., Chen, Y. H., Chen, H., Liu, Y. Y., & Wang, Y. X. (2011, January). The function of hypothalamus - pituitary - adrenal axis in children with ADHD. *Brain Research, 1368*, 159-162.

[163] Maidment, I. D. (2003). Efficacy of stimulants in adult ADHD. *Annals of Pharmacotherapy, 37*(12), 1884-1890.

[164] Mala, E. (2002). Hyperkineticke poruchy. *Pediatrie pro praxi, 1*, 14-17.

[165] Mala, E. (2008). ADHD – symptom a pohlavi. *Ceska a slovenska psychiatrie, 104*(4), 172–179.

[166] Manuck, S. B., Flory, J. D., Ferrell, R. E., Mann, J. J., & Muldoon, M. F. (2000). A regulatory polymorphism of the monoamine oxidase-A gene may be associated with variability in aggression, impulsivity, and central nervous system serotonergic responsivity. *Psychiatry Research, 95*(1), 9-23.

[167] Martaskova, D., Slachtova, L., Kemlink, D., Zahorakova, D., & Papezova, H. (2009). Polymorphisms in serotonin-related genes in anorexia nervosa. The first study in Czech population and metaanalyses with previously performed studies. *Folia Biologica, 55*(5), 192–197.

[168] Matejcek, Z. (2003). Poznamka k evolucnimu pohledu na syndrom ADHD. *Psychiatrie pro praxi, 3*, 131-133.

[169] Mattison, D. R., Plant, T. M., Lin, H. M., Chen, H. C., Chen, J. J., Twaddle, N. C., et al. (2011). Pubertal delay in male nonhuman primates (Macaca mulatta) treated with methylphenidate. *Proceedings of the National Academy of Sciences of the United States of America, 108*(39), 16301-16306.

[170] McGee, R., Birkbeck, J., & Silva, P. A. (1985). Physical development of hyperactive boys. *Developmental Medicine and Child Neurology, 27*(3), 364-368.

[171] McGough, J., McCracken, J., Swanson, J., Riddle, M., Kollins, S., Greenhill, L., et al. (2006). Pharmacogenetics of methylphenidate response in preschoolers with ADHD. *Journal of the American Academy of Child and Adolescent Psychiatry, 45*(11), 1314-1322.

[172] Michelson, D., Allen, A. J., Busner, J., Casat, C., Dunn, D., Kratochvil, C., et al. (2002). Once-daily atomoxetine treatment for children and adolescents with attention deficit hyperactivity disorder: a randomized, placebo-controlled study. *American Journal of Psychiatry, 159*(11), 1896–1901.

[173] Mick, E., Wozniak, J., Wilens, T. E., Biederman, J., & Faraone, S. V. (2009, February). Family-based association study of the BDNF, COMT and serotonin transporter genes and DSMIV bipolar-I disorder in children. *BioMed Central Psychiatry, 9*, 2-7.

[174] Mikami, A. Y., Hinshaw, S. P., Patterson, K. A., & Lee, J. C. (2008). Eating pathology among adolescent girls with attention-deficit/hyperactivity disorder. *Journal of Abnormal Psychology, 117*(1), 225–235.

[175] Miller, S. R., Miller, C. J., Bloom, J. S., Hynd, G. W., & Craggs, J. G. (2006, February). Right hemisphere brain morphology, attention-deficit hyperactivity disorder (ADHD) subtype, and social comprehension. *Journal of Child Neurology, 21*(2), 139-144.

[176] Millichap, J. G., (1978). Growth of Hyperactive Children Treated with Methylphenidate. *Journal of Learning Disabilities, 11*(9), 567-570.

[177] Millichap, J. G., & Millichap, M. (1975, June). Letter: Growth of hyperactive children. *The New England Journal of Medicine, 292*(24), 1300.

[178] Mills, S., Langley, K., Van den Bree, M., Street, E., Turic, D., Owen, M. J., et al. (2004, June). No evidence of association between Catechol-O-Methyltransferase (COMT) Val158Met genotype and performance on neuropsychological tasks in children with ADHD: A case-control study. *BioMed Central Psychiatry, 4*(1), 15-19.

[179] Molina, B. S., Hinshaw, S. P., Swanson, J. M., Arnold, L. E., Vitiello, B., Jensen, P. S., et al. (2009). The MTA at 8 years: prospective follow-up of children treated for combined-type ADHD in a multisite study. *Journal of the American Academy of Child and Adolescent Psychiatry, 48*(5), 484-500.

[180] Moon, D. S., Paik, J. W., Cho, A., Kim, J. W., Kim, E. J., & Chung, J. H. (2010). Association of schizophrenia and dopamine b-hydroxylase (DBH) polymorphism in Korean population. *European Neuropsychopharmacology 20*, 220–221.

[181] Mostofsky, S. H., Newschaffer, C. J., & Denckla, M. B. (2003). Overflow movements predict impaired response inhibition in children with ADHD. *Perceptual and Motor Skills, 97*(3), 1315-1331.

[182] Mostofsky, S. H., Wendlandt, J., Cutting, L., Denckla, M. B., & Singer, H. S. (1999), Corpus callosum measurements in girls with Tourette syndrome. *Neurology, 53*(6), 1345-1347.

[183] Moungnoi, F., & Maipang, P. (2011). Long-Term Effects of Short-Acting Methylphenidate on Growth Rates of Children with Attention

Deficit Hyperactivity Disorder at Queen Sirikit National Institute of Child Health. *Journal of the Medical Association of Thailand, 94*(3), 158-163.

[184] MTA Cooperative Group (2004). National Institute of Mental Health Multimodal Treatment Study of ADHD Follow-up: changes in effectiveness and growth after the end of treatment. *Pediatrics, 113*(4), 762–769.

[185] Muglia, P., Jain, U., & Kennedy, J. L. (2002). A transmission disequilibrium test of the Ser9/Gly dopamine D3 receptor gene polymorphism in adult attention-deficit hyperactivity disorder. *Behavioural Brain Research, 130*(1-2), 91-95.

[186] Munden, A., & Arcelus, J. (2002). *Poruchy pozornosti a hyperaktivita*. Praha: Portal, pp. 120.

[187] Murphy, K., & Barkley, R. A. (1996). Attention deficit hyperactivity disorder inadults: Comorbidities and adaptive impairments. *Comprehensive Psychiatry, 37*(6), 393-401.

[188] Mustillo, S., Worthman, C., Erkanli, A., Keller, G., Angold, A., & Costello, J. (2003, April). Obesity and Psychiatric disorder: Developmental Trajectories. *Pediatrics, 111*(1), 851-859.

[189] Nazar, B. P., Pinna, C. M., Coutinho, G., Segenreich, D., Duchesne, M., Appolinario, J. C., Mattos, P., et al. (2008, December). Review of literature of attention-deficit/hyperactivity disorder with comorbid eating disorders. *Revista Brasileira de Psiquiatria, 30*(4), 384-389.

[190] Nigg, J., Nikolas, M., Friderici, K., Park, L., & Zucker, R. A. (2007). Genotype and neuropsychological response inhibition as resilience promoters for attention-deficit/hyperactivity disorder, oppositional defiant disorder, and conduct disorder under conditions of psychosocial adversity. *Developmental and Psychopathology, 19*(3), 767-786.

[191] Nobile, M., Rusconi, M., Bellina, M., Marino, C., Giorda, R., Carlet, O., et al. (2009, November). COMT Val158Met polymorphism and socioeconomic status interact to predict attention deficit/hyperactivity problems in children aged 10-14. *European Child and Adolescent Psychiatry, 19*(7), 549-557.

[192] Ogdie, M. N., Fisher, S. E., Yang, M., Ishii, J., Francks, C., Loo, S. K., et al. (2004). Attention deficit hyperactivity disorder: fine mapping supports linkage to 5p13, 6q12, 16p13, and 17p11. *American Journal of Human Genetics, 75*(4), 661–668.

[193] Ogdie, M. N., Macphie, I. L., Minassian, S. L., Yang, M., Fisher, S. E., Francks, C., et al. (2003). A genomewide scan for attention-

deficit/hyperactivity disorder in an extended sample: suggestive linkage on 17p11. *American Journal of Human Genetics, 72*(5), 1268–1279.

[194] Ouellet-Morin, I., Wigg, K. G., Feng, Y., Dionne, G., Robaey, P., Brendgen, M., et al. (2008). Association of the dopamine transporter gene and ADHD symptoms in a Canadian population-based sample of same-age twins. *American Journal of Medical Genetics Part B, Neuropsychiatric Genetics, 147*(8), 1442–1449.

[195] Paclt, I. (2007). *Hyperkineticka porucha a poruchy chovani*. Praha: Grada.

[196] Paclt, I., & Florian, J. (1998). *Psychofarmakologie detskeho veku*. Praha: Grada.

[197] Paclt, I., Drtilkova, I., Kopeckova, M., Theiner, P., Sery, O., & Cermakova, N. (2010). The association between TaqI A polymorphism of ANKK1 (DRD2) gene and ADHD in the Czech boys aged between 6 and 13 years. *Neuro Endocrinology Letters, 31*(1), 131-136.

[198] Paclt, I., Koudelova, J., Pacltova, D., & Kopeckova, M. (2009). Dopamine beta hydroxylase (DBH) plasma activity in childhood mental disorders. *Neuroendocrinology Letters, 30*(5), 604-609.

[199] Paclt, I., Ptacek, R., & Florian, J. (2006). *Hyperaktivita*. Praha: Vzdelavaci institut ochrany deti.

[200] Pagoto, S. L., Curtin, C., Lemon, S. C., Bandini, L. G., Schneider, K. L., Bodenlos, J. S., et al. (2009). Association between adult attention deficit/hyperactivity disorder and obesity in the US population. *Obesity, 17*(3), 539–544.

[201] Papezova, H. (2006). Nove otazky a jejich reseni u poruch prijmu potravy. *Casopis lekaru ceskych, 145*(3), 181-183.

[202] Personen, A. K., Kajantie, E., Jones, A., Pyhälä, R., Lahti, J., Heinonen, K., et al. (2011, November). Symptoms of attention deficit hyperactivity disorder in children are associated with cortisol responses to psychosocial stress but not with daily cortisol levels. *Journal of Psychiatric Research, 45*(11), 1471-1476.

[203] Pliszka, S. R., Matthews, T. L., Braslow, K. J., & Watson, M. A. (2006). Comparative effects of methylphenidate and mixed salts amphetamine on height and weight in children with attention-deficit/hyperactivity disorder. *Journal of the American Academy of Child and Adolescent Psychiatry, 45*(5), 520-526.

[204] Polanczyk, G., Zeni, C., Genro, J. P., Guimarães, A. P., Roman, T., Hutz, M. H., et al. (2007, February). Association of the adrenergic alpha2A receptor gene with methylphenidate improvement of

inattentive symptoms in children and adolescents with attention-deficit/hyperactivity disorder. *Archives of General Psychiatry, 64*(2), 218-224.

[205] Pomerleau, O. F., Downey, K. K., Stelson, F. W., & Pomerleau, C. S. (1995). Cigarette smoking in adult patients diagnosed with attention deficit hyperactivity disorder. *Journal of Substance Abuse Treatment, 7*(3), 373-378.

[206] Poulton, A. (2005). Growth on stimulant medication; clarifying the confusion: a review. *Archives of Disease in Childhood, 90*(8), 801-806.

[207] Poulton, A., & Cowell, C. T. (2003). Slowing of growth in height and weight on stimulants: a characteristic pattern. *Journal of Paediatrics and Child Health, 39*(3), 180-185.

[208] Poulton, A., & Nanan, R. (2009, May). Stimulant medications and growth. *Journal of the American Academy of Child and Adolescent Psychiatry, 48*(5), 574-576.

[209] Prince, J. (2008, June). Catecholamine dysfunction in attention-deficit/hyperactivity disorder: an update. *Journal of Clinical Psychopharmacology, 28*(2), 39-45.

[210] Ptacek, R., & Kuzelova, H. (2010). ADHD – variabilita v dětství a dospělosti [ADHD – variability in childhood and adulthood]. Praha: Karolinum.

[211] Ptacek, R., Kuzelova, H., & Paclt, I. (2009b). ADHD and growth: Anthropometric changes in medicated and non-medicated ADHD boys. *Medical Science Monitor, 15*(12), 595-599.

[212] Ptacek, R., Kuzelova, H., Paclt, I., & Zukov, I. (2008). Vliv medikace na antropometrické charakteristiky dětí s ADHD. *Ceska a slovenska Psychiatrie, 104*(8), 415-419.

[213] Ptacek, R., Kuzelova, H., Paclt, I., Zukov, I., & Fischer, S. (2009a). Somatic and Endocrinological Changes in non Medicated ADHD Children. *Prague Medical Report, 110*(1), 25–34.

[214] Ptacek, R., Kuzelova, H., Paclt, I., Zukov, I., & Fischer, S. (2009c). Anthropometric changes in nonmedicated ADHD boys. *Neuro Endocrinology Letters, 30*(3), 377-381.

[215] Purdie, N., Hattie, J., & Carroll, A. (2002). A Review of the Research on Interventions for Attention-Deficit Hyperactivity Disorder: What Works Best? *Review of Educational Research, 72*(1), 61–99.

[216] Purper-Ouakil, D., Wohl, M., Mouren, M. C., Verpillat, P., Ades, J., & Gorwood, P. (2005). Meta-analysis of family-based association studies

between the dopamine transporter gene and attention deficit hyperactivity disorder. *Psychiatric Genetics, 15*(1), 53-59.

[217] Purper-Ouakil, D., Wohl, M., Orejarena, S., Cortese, S., Boni, C., Asch, M., et al. (2008, December). Pharmacogenetics of methylphenidate response in attention deficit/hyperactivity disorder: association with the dopamine transporter gene (SLC6A3). *American Journal of Medical Genetics Part B, Neuropsychiatric Genetics, 147*(8), 1425-1430.

[218] Quist, J. F., Barr, C. L., Schachar, R., Roberts, W., Malone, M., Tannock, R., et al. (2003). The serotonin 5-HT1B receptor gene and attention deficit hyperactivity disorder. *Molecular Psychiatry, 8*(1), 98–102.

[219] Rao, J. K., Julius, J. R., Breen, T. J., & Blethen, S. L. (1998). Response to Growth Hormone in Attention Deficit Hyperactivity Disorder: Effects of Methylphenidate and Pe-moline Therapy. *Pediatrics, 102*(3), 497-500.

[220] Reda, M. M., & El-Hadidy, E. (2011). Serum leptin in children with attention deficit hyperactivity disorder. *Middle East Current Psychiatry, 18*(1), 1-5.

[221] Roman, T., Polanczyk, G. V., Zeni, C., Genro, J. P., Rohde, L. A., & Hutz, M. H. (2006). Further evidence of the involvement of alpha-2A-adrenergic receptor gene (ADRA2A) in inattentive dimensional scores of attention-deficit/hyperactivity disorder. *Molecular Psychiatry, 11*(1), 8–10.

[222] Roman, T., Schmitz, M., Polanczyk, G. V., Eizirik, M., Rohde, L. A., & Hutz, M. H. (2003). Is the alpha-2A adrenergic receptor gene (ADRA2A) associated with attentiondeficit/ hyperactivity disorder? *American Journal of Medical Genetics Part B, Neuropsychiatric Genetics, 120*(1), 116–120.

[223] Roman, T., Szobot, C., Martins, S., Biederman, J., Rohde, L. A., & Hutz, M. H. (2002, August). Dopamine transporter gene and response to methylphenidate in attention-deficit/hyperactivity disorder. *Pharmacogenetics, 12*(6), 497-499.

[224] Romanos, M., Freitag, C., Jacob, C., Craig, D. W., Dempfle, A., Nquen, T. T., et al. (2008). Genome-wide linkage analysis of ADHD using high-density SNP arrays: novel loci at 5q13.1 and 14q12. *Molecular Psychiatry, 13*(5), 522–530.

[225] Rose, S. R., Reeves, G., Gut, R., & Germak, J. (2011). Impact of Attention Deficit Hyperactivity Disorder (ADHD) Treatment on Response to Growth Hormone Therapy (GHT). *Pediatric Academic*

Societies (PAS) and Asian Society for Pediatric Research 2011 Annual Meeting: Abstract 1402.24. Presented April 30, 2011.

[226] Rubia, K., Cubillo, A., Woolley, J., Brammer, M. J., & Smith, A. (2011, April). Disorder-specific dysfunctions in patients with attention-deficit/hyperactivity disorder compared to patients with obsessive-compulsive disorder during interference inhibition and attention allocation. *Human Brain Mapping, 32*(4), 601-611.

[227] Safer, D. J., & Allen, R. P. (1973). Factors influencing the suppressant effects of two stimulant drugs on the growth of hyperactive children. *Pediatrics, 51*(4), 660–667.

[228] Safer, D. J., Allen, R. P., & Barr, E. (1972). Depression of growth in hyperactive children on stimulant drugs. *The New England Journal of Medicine, 287*(5), 217-220.

[229] Sagvolden, T., Russell, V. A., Aase, H., Johansen, E. B., & Farshbaf, M. (2005). Rodent models of attention-deficit/hyperactivity disorder. *Biological Psychiatry, 57*(11), 1239–1247.

[230] Sales, A. (2000). 'Substance Abuse and Disability', Substance Abuse and Counseling. A Perspective. ERIC document reproduction service, no. 440352.

[231] Schertz, M., Adesman, A. R., Alfieri, N. E., & Bienkowski, R. S. (1996). Predictors of weight loss in children with attention deficit hyperactivity disorder treated with stimulant medi-cation. *Pediatrics, 98*(4), 763-769.

[232] Schmitz, M., Denardin, D., Silva, T. L., Pianca, T., Roman, T., Hutz, M. H., et al. (2006, November). Association between alpha-2a-adrenergic receptor gene and ADHD inattentive type. *Biological Psychiatry, 60*(10), 1028-1033.

[233] Schoechlin, C., & Engel, R. R. (2005). Neuropsychological performance in adult attention-deficit hyperactivity disorder: Meta-analysis of empirical data. *Archives of Clinical Neuropsychology, 20*(6), 727-744.

[234] Seeger, G., Schloss, P., & Schmidt, M. H. (2001). Marker gene polymorphisms in hyperkinetic disorder: predictors of clinical response to treatment with methylphenidate? *Neuroscience Letters, 313*(1-2), 45-48.

[235] Setoodeh, A., & Teleffson, S. (2007). Attention Deficit Hyperactivity Disorder and Growth. *Iranian Journal od Pediatrics, 17*(2), 183-187.

[236] Shaw, P., & Rabin, C. (2009). New insights into attention-deficit/hyperactivity disorder using structural neuroimaging. *Current Psychiatry Reports, 11*(5), 393-398.

[237] Shaw, P., Eckstrand, K., Sharp, W., Blumenthal, J., Lerch, J. P., Greenstein, D., et al. (2007). Attention-deficit/hyperaktivity disorder is characterized by a delay in cortical maturation. *Proceeding ot the National Academy Sciences United States of America, 104*(49), 19649-19654.

[238] Shaw, P., Lerch, J., Greenstein, D., Sharp, W., Clasen, L., Evans, A., et al. (2006). Longitudinal mapping of cortical thickness and clinical outcome in children and adolescents with attention-deficit/hyperactivity disorder. *Archives of General Psychiatry, 63*(5), 540-549.

[239] Sheehan, K., Lowe, N., Kirley, A., Mullins, C., Fitzgerald, M., Gill, M., et al. (2005). Tryptophan hydroxylase 2 (TPH2) gene variants associated with ADHD. *Molecular Psychiatry, 10*(10), 944–949.

[240] Silk, T. J., Vance, A., Rinehart, N., Bradshaw, J. L., & Cunnington, R. (2009). White-matter abnormalities in attention deficit hyperactivity disorder: A diffusion tensor imaging study. *Human Brain Mapping, 30*(9), 2757-2765.

[241] Sinn, N., & Bryan, J. (2007, April). Effect of supplementation with polyunsaturated fatty acids and micronutrients on learning and behavior problems associated with child ADHD. *Journal of Develepmental and Behavioral Pediatrics, 28*(2), 82-91.

[242] Smahel, Z. (2001). *Principy teorie a metody auxologie.* Praha: Karolinum.

[243] Smith, B. H., Molina, B. S. G., & Pelham, W. E. (2002). The clinically meaningful link between alcohol and attention-deficit/hyperactivity disorder. *Alcohol, Health, and Research World, 26*(2), 122–129.

[244] Smoller, J. W., Biederman, J., Arbeitman, L., Doyle, A. E., Fagerness, J., Perlis, R. H., et al. (2006). Association between the 5HT1B receptor gene (HTR1B) and the inattentive subtype of ADHD. *Biological Psychiatry, 59*(5), 460–467.

[245] Solanto, M. V., Arnsten, A. F. T. & Castellanos, F. X. (2001). The Neuroscience of Stimulant Drug Action in ADHD. In M. V. Solanto, A. F. T. Arnsten & F. X. Castellanos, *Stimulant Drugs and ADHD: Basic and Clinical Neuroscience* (pp. 355-379). New York: Oxford University Press.

[246] Soldin, O. P., Nandedkar, A. K., Japal, K. M., Stein, M., Mosee, S., Magrab, P., et al. (2002, May). Newborn thyroxine levels and childhood ADHD. *Clinical Biochemistry, 35*(2), 131-136.

[247] Spencer, T., Biederman, J., & Wilens, T. (1998). Growth deficits in children with attention deficit hyperactivity disorder. *Pediatrics, 102*(3), 501-506.

[248] Spencer, T. J., Biederman, J., Wilens, T., Guite, J., & Harding, M. (1995, July). ADHD and thyroid abnormalities: a research note. *Journal of Child Psychology and Psychiatry, 36*(5), 879-885.

[249] Spencer, T. J., Faraone, S. V., Biederman, J., Lerner, M., Cooper, K. M., & Zimmerman, B. (2006, May). Concerta Study Group. Does prolonged therapy with a long-acting stimulant suppress growth in children with ADHD? *Journal of American Academy of Child and Adolescent Psychiatry, 45*(5), 527-537.

[250] Spencer, T. J., Heiligenstein, J. H., Biederman, J., Faries, D. E., Kratochvil, C. J., Conners, C. K., et al. (2002). Results from 2 proof-of-concept, placebo-controlled studies of atomoxetine in children with attention-deficit/hyperaktivity disorder. *Journal of Clinical Psychiatry, 63*(12), 1140–1147.

[251] Stadler, C., Kroeger, A., Weyers, P., Grasmann, D., Horschinek, M., Freitag, C., et al. (2011, May). Cortisol reactivity in boys with attention-deficit/hyperactivity disorder and disruptive behavior problems: the impact of callous unemotional traits. *Psychiatry Research, 187*(1-2), 204-209.

[252] Stark, R., Bauer, E., Merz, C. J., Zimmermann, M., Reuter, M., Plichta, M. M., et al. (2011, February). ADHD related behaviors are associated with brain activation in the reward system. *Neuropsychologia, 49*(3), 426-434.

[253] Stein, M. A., & Weiss, R. E. (2003, April). Thyroid function tests and neurocognitive functioning in children referred for attention deficit/hyperactivity disorder. *Psychoneuroendocrinology, 28*(3), 304-316.

[254] Stein, M. A., Waldman, I. D., Sarampote, C. S., Seymour, K. E., Robb, A. S., Conlone, C., et al. (2005, July). Dopamine transporter genotype and methylphenidate dose response in children with ADHD. *Neuropsychopharmacology, 30*(7), 1374-1382.

[255] Sterman, M. B. (2000). EEG Markers for Attention Deficit Disorder: Pharmacological and Neurofeedback Applications. *Child Study Journal, 30*(1), 1–24.

[256] Stevenson, J. (1992). Evidence for a genetic etiology in hyperaktivity in children. *Behavior Genetic, 22*, 337-344.

[257] Still, G. F. (1902). Some abnormal psychical conditions in children: the Goulstonian lectures. *The Lancet, 1*, 1008–1012.

[258] Strauss, A. A., & Lehtinen, L. E. (1947). *Psychopathology and education of the brain-injured child*. New York: Grune and Stratton.

[259] Strimas, R., Davis, C., Patte, K., Curtis, C., Reid, C., & McCool, C. (2008). Symptoms of attention-deficit/hyperactivity disorder, overeating, and body mass index in men. *Eating Behaviors, 9*(4), 516-518.

[260] Sund, A. M., & Zeiner, P. (2002). Does extended medication with amphetamine or methylphenidate reduce growth in hyperactive children? *Nordic Journal of Psychiatry, 56*(1), 53–57.

[261] Surman, C. B., Randall, E. T., & Biederman, J. (2006). Association between attention-deficit/hyperactivity disorder and bulimia nervosa: analysis of 4 case-control studies. *Journal of Clinical Psychiatry, 67*(3), 351–354.

[262] Swanson, J., Greenhill, L. L., Wigal, T., Kollins, S. H., Stehli-Nguyen, A., Davies, M., et al. (2006). Stimulant-Related Reductions of Growth Rates in the PATS. *Journal of the American Academy of Child and Adolescent Psychiatry, 45*(11), 1304-1313.

[263] Swanson, J. M., Sergeant, J. A., Taylor, E., Sonuga-Barke, E. J. S., Jensen, P. S., & Cantwell, D. P. (1998). Attention-deficit Hyperactivity Disorder and Hyperkinetic Disorder. *The Lancet, 351*(9100), 429-433.

[264] Thapar, A., Cooper, M., Eyre, O., & Langley, K. (2013). Practitioner Review: What have we learnt about the causes of ADHD?. *Journal of Child Psychology and Psychiatry, 54*(1), 3-16.

[265] Tharoor, H., Lobos, E. A., Todd, R. D., & Reiersen, A. M. (2008, June). Association of dopamine, serotonin, and nicotinic gene polymorphisms with methylphenidate response in ADHD. *American Journal of Medical Genetics Part B, Neuropsychiatric Genetics, 147*(4), 527-530.

[266] Toren, P., Karasik, A., Eldar, S., Wolmer, L., Shimon, I., Weitz, R., et al. (1997, May-June). Thyroid function in attention deficit and hyperactivity disorder. *Journal of Psychiatric Research, 31*(3), 359-363.

[267] Vagnerova, M. (2001). *Kognitivni a socialni psychologie zaka zakladni skoly*. Praha: Karolinum.

[268] Vagnerova, M. (2005). *Vyvojova psychologie I.* Praha: Karolinum.

[269] Van West, D., Claes, S., & Deboutte, D. (2009). Differences in hypothalamic-pituitary–adrenal axis functioning among children with ADHD predominantly inattentive and combined types. *European Child and Adolescent Psychiatry, 18*(9), 543–553.

[270] Viggiano, D., Grammatikopoulos, G., & Sadile, A. G. (2002, March). A morphometric evidence for a hyperfunctioning mesolimbic system in an animal model of ADHD. *Behavioural Brain Research, 130*(1-2), 181-189.

[271] Vincent, J., Varley, C. K., & Leger, P. (1990). Effects of methylphenidate on early adolescent growth. *The American Journal of Psychiatry, 147*(4), 501-502.

[272] Volkow, N. D., Wang, G. J., Fowler, J. S., & Ding, Y. S. (2005). Imaging the effects of methylphenidate on brain dopamine: new model on its therapeutic actions for attention-deficit/hyperactivity disorder. *Biological Psychiatry, 57*(11), 1410-1415.

[273] von Ranson, K. M., & Cassin, S. E. (2007). Eating disorders and addiction: Theory and evidence. In J. S. Rubin (Ed.), *Eating Disorders and Weight Loss Research* (pp. 1-37). New York: Nova Science Publishers.

[274] Walitza, S., Renner, T. J., Dempfle, A., Konrad, K.,Wewetzer, C., Halbach, A., et al. (2005). Transmission disequilibrium of polymorphic variants in the tryptofan hydroxylase-2 gene in attention-deficit/hyperactivity disorder. *Molecular Psychiatry, 10*(12), 1126–1132.

[275] Waring, M. E., & Lapane, K. L. (2008). Overweight in Children and Adolescents in Relation to Attention-Deficit/Hyperactivity Disorder: Results From a National Sample. *Pediatrics, 122*(1), 1-6.

[276] Waxman, S. E. (2009, November). A systematic review of impulsivity in eating disorders. *European Eating Disorders Review, 17*(6), 408-425.

[277] Webster-Stratton, C., Reid, M. J., & Hammond, M. (2001). Social skills and problem solving training for children with early-onset conduct problems: who benefits? *Journal of Child Psychology and Psychiatry, 42*(7), 943–952.

[278] Weiss, R. E., Stein, M. A., Trommer, B., & Refetoff, S. (1993, October). Attention-deficit hyperactivity disorder and thyroid function. *Journal of Pediatrics, 123*(4), 539-545.

[279] Wilens, T. E. (2008). Effects of methylphenidate on the catecholaminergic system in attention-deficit/hyperactivity disorder. *Journal of Clinical Psychopharmacology, 28*(2), 46-53.

[280] Winsberg, B. G., & Comings, D. E. (1999, December). Association of the dopamine transporter gene (DAT1) with poor methylphenidate response. *Journal of the American Academy of Child and Adolescent Psychiatry, 38*(12), 1474-1477.

[281] Yan, T., McQuillin, A., Thapar, A., Asherson, P., Hunt, S., Stanford, S., et al. (2010, January). NK1 (TACR1) receptor gene 'knockout' mouse phenotype predicts genetic association with ADHD. *Journal of Psychopharmacology, 24*(1), 27-38.

[282] Yang, L., Wang, Y. F., Li, J., & Faraone, S. V. (2004, September). Association of norepinephrine transporter gene with methylphenidate response. *Journal of the American Academy of Child and Adolescent Psychiatry, 43*(9), 1154-1158.

[283] Zachor, D. A., Roberts, A. W., Hodgens, J. B., Isaacs, J. S., & Merrick, J. (2006). Effect of longterm psychostimulant medication on growth of children with ADHD. *Research of Deve-lopmental Disabilities, 27*(2), 162-174.

[284] Zametkin, A. J., Nordahl, T. E., Gross, M., King, A. C., Semple, W. E., Rumsey, J., et al. (1990). Cerebral glucose metabolism in adults with hyperactivity of childhood onset. *The New England Journal of Medicine, 323*(20), 1361-1366.

[285] Zametkin, A. J., Rapoport, J. L., Murphy, D. L., Linnoila, M., & Ismond, D. (1985). Treatment of hyperactive children with monoamine oxidase inhibitors. I. Clinical efficacy. *Archives of General Psychiatry, 42*(10), 962–966.

[286] Zeni, C. P., Guimaraes, A. P., Polanczyk, G. V., Genro, J. P., Roman, T., Hutz, M. H., et al. (2007, April). No signifiant association between response to methylphenidate and genes of the dopaminergic and serotonergic systems in a sample of Brazilian children with attention-deficit/ hyperactivity disorder. *American Journal of Medical Genetics Part B, Neuropsychiatric Genetics, 144*(3), 391-394.

[287] Zhang, H., Du, M., Zhuang, S., & Liu, M. (2005). Influence of methylphenidate on growth of school age children with attention deficit hyperactivity disorder. *Zhonghua Er Ke Za Zhi, 43*(10), 723-725.

[288] Zhou, K., Dempfle, A., Arcos-Burgos, M., Bakker, S. C., Banaschewski, T., Biederman, J., et al. (2008b). Meta-analysis of genome-wide linkage scans of attention deficit hyperactivity disorder. *American Journal of Medical Genetics Part B, Neuropsychiatric Genetics, 147*(8), 1392–1398.

[289] Zhou, K., Chen, W., Buitelaar, J., Banaschewski, T., Oades, R. D., Franke, B., et al. (2008a). Genetic heterogeneity in ADHD: DAT1 gene only affects probands without CD. *American Journal of Medical Genetics Part B, Neuropsychiatric Genetics, 147*(8), 1481–1487.

Index

D

E

F

G

H

I

K

L

M

N

O

P

Q

R

S

T

U

V

W

X

Y